JELLY BELLY

DR APARNA SANTHANAM is one of India's leading dermatologists and wellness experts, having worked in the field for over 15 years. She runs her own practice in Mumbai, apart from working as a strategic consultant to some of India's prominent wellness and beauty brands. She is also closely associated with Apnalaya, an organization that works on integrated community development of the most marginalized urban-poor.

Dr Santhanam believes in the principles of knowledge, prevention, moderation and protection when it comes to health, beauty and wellness. Having authored two books, *Skin Deep* and *Let's Talk Hair*, and worked with women across the socio-economic spectrum, she believes educating women about their own wellness needs and providing tools to access better health is the key to not just more healthy women, but to creating stronger families and communities as a whole.

Praise for *Skin Deep*

'A refreshing new look at skincare.' – *Indian Express*

'A must-read.' – *Afternoon Despatch & Courier*

'Grab a copy if you too want your skin to glow, naturally.' – *Mid Day*

Praise for *Let's Talk Hair*

'*Let's Talk Hair* offers recipes to help you get super-healthy hair, tests to assess the quality and type of your hair and scalp, and guidance on choosing the best products for your tresses. Hair and skin specialist Aparna Santhanam helps you get the kind of hair you've always wanted.' – *The Hindu*

'*Let's Talk Hair* provides everything you need to know to care for your crowning glory, from important lifestyle advice to simple hair care tips. From a basic understanding of hair, its growth and behaviour pattern through the various stages of its life, this book throws light on specific hair problems and how to tackle these effectively. *Let's Talk Hair* captures every aspect of hair care from oiling, cleansing and conditioning treatments to cutting, colouring and styling. It also offers advice on various haircare products, tells you how to eat right for those perfect tresses and also busts some commonly held beliefs and myths about coconut hair oil.' – *The Times of India*

JELLY BELLY

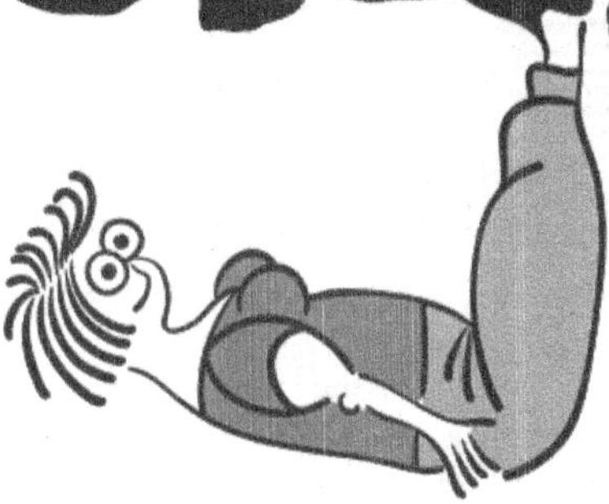

Every Woman's Guide to Good Health and Happiness

DR APARNA SANTHANAM

Collins

First published in India in 2015 by Collins
An imprint of HarperCollins *Publishers*
4th Floor, Tower A, Building No. 10, Phase II,
DLF Cyber City, Gurugram, Haryana -122002
www.harpercollins.co.in

P-ISBN: 978-93-5177-089-3
E-ISBN: 978-93-5177-090-9

2 4 6 8 10 9 7 5 3 1

Typeset in 11.5/14.5 Adobe Garamond Pro at
SÜRYA

Printed and bound at
Manipal Technologies Ltd., Manipal

To all the wonderful women who have touched my life, inspired and influenced me.

Contents

Introduction

Life today in India's metros is a race against time. Work lives seem accelerated with more and more men and women well-settled in their careers by their late 20s and early 30s. Conversely, personal lives seem to be on hold and the notion of 'settling down' seems to happen mainly in the late 20s and early 30s. The mid-30s is a good phase in many ways for women: the pressures of teenage are over, so is the drama of the 20s—the whole dating scene, the early trials of building a home, career, etc. Life settles to a happy pace, you are your own woman: content, yet raring to go and achieving your goals. From a health perspective, the body is still young and chuffing along just fine and you barely give any thought to the 35—except for the fact that you have hit the number! At 45-plus, there is an acceptance that creeps in, to some happily, to others reluctantly, that the body is going to display some signs of wear and tear—evidence of the life lived. Once 50 becomes a reality, one doesn't feel that old any more! People are still young, energetic and full of life.

But in the 35-plus decade, most women do not want to acknowledge the hiccups and hurdles they experience, pushing aside all thoughts of the passing years and determined to look away from the ticking clock. A host of things could happen to them. The list looks something like this:

- ❑ She goes to a party and someone says to her face that she has grown fat. People are free with their insults even though they say they are being her friend. She mutters under her breath: hell, they're just jealous of me.
- ❑ She's exhausted after climbing two flights of stairs. She thinks: but that building has really steep stairs.
- ❑ There are mornings when her face looks really tired even after a full night's sleep. She muses: it's time to change that pillow.
- ❑ She keeps popping paracetamol tablets a couple of times a week, for just a mild headache, you know—there's nothing really wrong with that, is there?
- ❑ Suddenly, the first day of the periods is killing, but could it be because she's stressing herself too much?
- ❑ Wearing heels is no longer fun. The lower back hurts a little, and so do the knees. But then, who needs heels anyway?
- ❑ She is tired of watching what she eats all the time. Why can't she just eat healthy and stop worrying about her weight?

There are plenty more in the master list that I have gleaned from my friends and patients over the years, all of which have pointed me to the conclusion that at 35-plus, women, who are not yet middle aged nor ill, just want to continue wearing their heels and feeling good about themselves. They do wish sometimes that someone would give them that magic pill that would make them energetic and ready to deal with the millions of chores and duties while also finding a little time for themselves.

About a year ago, a patient of mine, Devaki, visited me. Devaki had first consulted me about five years back. She was 32 and had had a bad outbreak of a skin allergy, and I had treated her successfully then. We had struck up an instant friendship. We stayed in touch and called each other on birthdays and anniversaries. She would swing by the clinic once in a while, but I had not seen her in a couple of years. When we eventually met for coffee, I noticed that she looked a bit tired. So I asked her what was wrong. And that just opened up the proverbial floodgates!

'Nothing, everything,' she said. 'I just feel like I'm riding on a non-stop roller-coaster where I keep doing things and yet always have more things to do. I feel like my "to-do list" is endless. Drop the kids to school, organize their classes, stay on top of my work, take my mom for her physiotherapy, organize meals with the cook according to each one's preferences, visit my in-laws once a fortnight … the list is endless and I just don't have the energy for all this! I get angry with everyone, especially my kids, all the time; I hate myself for being an angry parent, but I cannot control it. On top of that, I recently consulted my family doctor about this funny heel pain I've been having, but both the doctor and my husband think that I am just asking for attention.'

Devaki's situation, I realized, was an all too familiar one. I have heard various women express similar angst with their lives, but it had just never struck home so forcefully before. This one conversation was illuminating for me in terms of realizing what my patients, I myself and, no doubt, countless other women, deal with on a daily basis.

So I decided to put together all the non-specific 'non-problems' that 35-plus women experience, and identify the patterns and offer solutions that are doable. Some of these problems are truly physical, although their expressions may be psychological or emotional. 35-plus women are beautiful, secure, confident and in control of themselves for the most part. And I truly believe that they should not allow the niggling irritants to diminish the beauty of this phase of their lives.

I've tried to cover the most common issues related to their health and well-being at this magical yet difficult stage, but this by no means is an exhaustive list. Also, this book is not a substitute for a doctor or a health care provider's role in any way. It is intended to make women more aware of their bodies and more mindful of the factors they can bring under their control.

The pressures of trying to successfully hold down a career, home, kids, husband, extended family and friends is cause for a number of stress-related illnesses that are plaguing women across the country. In the crazy mix of trying to keep the home-work balance perfect, women often forget to take care of themselves. A study done four years ago in the UK has shown that among the four groups, married men, single men, married women and single women, the category that is the healthiest and happiest is married men, followed by single women, followed by single men and the poorest health, sadly, is among married women. A recent study from Harvard showed that men benefit more from marriage healthwise than women. In India, at least from what I see, the situation is even more skewed. It is fairly evident that when life gets busy, women with families to look after neglect their own needs. Prolonged periods of neglect lead to poor health and well-being and, sometimes, a complete psychological breakdown.

This book has only one lesson for you, dear reader: be kind to your body, treat it as your temple, and nourish it with goodness. Whether you are single, married, divorced or anything in-between, remember that it is up to you to take charge of your health and well-being.

Good health is the cornerstone of a fulfilling and happy existence. A niggle here, a twinge there can often not just mar your day, but develop into full-blown issues if not nipped in the bud. So read on and find your own path to a healthy, productive and essentially happy life!

1

The Four Cornerstones of Health and Happiness

Before we look closely at many of the common ailments that plague women above 35, I want to share with you a few simple, scientifically proven truths. The quest for a healthy existence is as old as civilization itself and ancient systems of healing have been practised for centuries across the world. While a lot of modern medicine is about diagnosis and treatment, in recent years the focus has slowly but surely shifted to prevention. Also, modern medicine has subtly become more participative and less prescriptive.

Active participation from all of us, as patients, definitely delivers better outcomes on health and happiness. However, to be active participants driving one's own health and well-being, there are four lifestyle choices that I consider absolutely essential: Learn Right, Eat Smart, Move To Improve and Stress Release.

1. LEARN RIGHT: *Acquire reliable information and knowledge about health issues*—The first step towards

understanding health is through trustworthy information and knowledge about health issues one may face. And that knowledge is two-pronged: knowledge about your own body, and knowledge about age-related health issues and their preventive care. So, in a world of information overload, how can you ensure that you are getting accurate and correct information?

a. The best way to procure the correct information is by asking your doctor. Your general or primary health care physician is the most dependable guide on issues that you might potentially have to watch out for. Before you make an appointment, write down the questions that you would like to ask your doctor on a piece of paper and ensure you get enough time with him or her to get all the answers you need.
b. Look for reliable sources of information like websites run by medical colleges of repute, health clinics, etc. Do *not* believe every Internet site you may stumble on to. Many of them survive through creating shock effects in the minds of readers and are likely to spook you out instead of being a help.

2. EAT SMART: *Focus on nutrition*—Good health is largely dependent on good nutrition; many physical and emotional ailments can be traced back to a diet deficient in vitamins and minerals. Food is the primary source of nutrition. Many medicines designed to improve the health contain synthetic replicas of enzymes and chemicals found in nutrient-dense foods, but you should not take these supplements unless absolutely necessary. A well-balanced diet can lower the incidence of disease,

help in quicker recovery from illnesses and improve both the quality and the length of life. In contrast, inadequate nutrition and poor-quality foods generally reduce the life span of an individual and can make him or her the victim of various deformities and diseases.

The body needs energy for metabolism, for elimination of wastes, and for execution of its immune, digestive, cardiovascular, nervous and respiratory systems. Individual parts of the body rely on specific nutrients for their growth. For example, the brain depends on carbohydrates, fatty acids, iron, iodine and Vitamin-B12 to function with clarity and efficiency. Bone health depends on calcium and Vitamin-D3. Protein and potassium are some of the nutrients that fuel muscle health. Enough fibre in the diet can greatly reduce the chances of constipation, colon cancer and haemorrhoids; some fibrous foods would be green vegetables, oats and legumes, which enable the colon to function efficiently.

A balanced diet can usually provide all the nutrition necessary to excel at most daily activities. Daily needs for women include four to six servings of fruits and vegetables, three to four servings of protein, and some complex carbohydrates along with nuts and legumes. At least two servings of dairy or dairy substitutes are also highly recommended. Although this, at first glance, seems like a lot of food, it is not! One egg is a serving of protein as is four pieces of paneer, half an apple is one serving of fruit, one chapatti is a serving of carbohydrates, a cup of dal is a serving of carbohydrate and protein.

Nuts can be eaten quite generously as also sprouts and legumes, and they provide protein, fibre and carbohydrates.

A smart way to ensure good health is to plan your meals in advance. A general rule that can be followed is to eat one protein like eggs, one dairy, one fruit and one fibre-based cereal like oats for breakfast. For lunch, one can eat one protein, one complex carbohydrate and two to three servings of vegetables with one serving of dairy. Two vegetables and a large helping of salad at dinner, along with one protein and one grain, can cap the day and deliver all the required nutrition.

Healthy eating helps to maintain consistent weight and BMI control, and fosters a sense of health and happiness.

3. MOVE TO IMPROVE: *Exercise regularly*—The old adage 'move to improve' has never been truer than today. Most middle and upper middle-class women lead sedentary lives without realizing how injurious it is to the health. Exercise boosts energy, helps control weight, releases happiness hormones, and enables one to sleep better. Exercise can help you relax and promote a sense of well-being.

   You should do at least 30 minutes of high-intensity aerobic activity for at least five days a week, coupled with muscle-strengthening exercises to work all the muscle groups at least twice a week. Walking briskly, running, cycling, playing a sport – you can choose any of the aerobic options, while for muscle strengthening you would need to do yoga, Pilates or work out at the gym under the supervision of a trainer.

4. STRESS RELEASE: *Care for your emotional well-being*—Once we have looked at the structural, nutritional and physical aspects of health, it is also important to look at one's state of emotional well-being. It is necessary to have a sense of satisfaction in relationships, comfort in the work place, adequate rest and holiday breaks to keep the mind healthy. Very often, emotional stress triggers various lifestyle conditions and delays healing. Women, in particular, tend to suppress stress and express it as physical ailments, unknown to themselves, and it is therefore important to be aware of it.

   Emotional well-being and mental health concerns are major health issues in their own right. And they can also greatly affect physical health. Stress, depression, anxiety can weaken the immune system and lead to a host of ailments like digestive disorders, irregular periods, headaches and fever. The challenge is two-pronged: treat the mind while simultaneously caring for the body.

   Emotions that are affirmative are life-generating–they inspire joy, creativity and helps to recover from physical ailments. Positive attitudes such as peace, gratitude, awe, love, interest, serenity and feeling connected to others directly impact one's health and well-being. But it is also up to us to develop these emotions.

Having understood the four cornerstones, let us now look at the different conditions and ailments that may detract from our sense of well-being.

2

Testing Times

We all groan at the mention of the word *test.* Why do we need to do it? Aren't our lives too full anyway? When do we have the time to go to the doctor and do tests when we are feeling just fine? It is so unnecessary, such a waste of time and money.

Well, the truth is: it is not! There is enough scientific research to show that regular screening for lifestyle conditions and other disorders actually promotes better health. Preventive health care is the best way to insure against diseases and so diagnostic screening tests are a must, especially for women above 35. Often these tests will detect deviations or anomalies that were not obvious otherwise. The old adage, 'prevention is better than cure' is more true for health care than any other field.

But what should one test?

While there are many ways of dividing these tests–by condition, by speciality, etc., I am going to list the different tests that must be done according to age.

Screening Tests for the Woman in Her 30s

This is the decade when you should watch out for the early warning signals. Many of you will be having babies in this age, and may be paying attention solely to those parts of your anatomy. Some of you may be already past child-bearing and have long since forgotten that you must take care of yourself. If you are focused on your career, maybe you are relying on the office vending machine for your tea or coffee and often don't have the energy to shop or eat healthy. That effortless metabolism of a decade ago seems a distant past.

The thirties is the decade of slowing down of body mechanisms but revving up the pace of life in general. And often, this creates imbalances in the body that may develop into more complex issues later on in life. Testing will help you to flag up these issues so that you know what precautions to take.

Full Gynaecological Check

Your gynaecologist will perform manual pelvic and breast examinations, plus a pap smear (during which cervical cells are collected with a swab).

Why do you need it? A pelvic exam checks for abnormalities such as growths. A breast exam will identify any suspicious lumps, dimpling, rashes and nipple discharge. And the pap smear is an important screening for cervical cancer.

How often do you need it? All women thirty and older need annual pelvic exams (a breast exam is typically included). The exception: You may be able to skip a year or two if three consecutive, annual pap tests show normal results.

Tip: For the most accurate pap results, avoid having sex or using vaginal medications (such as anti-yeast creams) one to two days before your appointment.

At home perform monthly breast self-examinations (manual checks for lumps), despite debate about whether these exams help prevent breast cancer deaths. Do it about a week after you start your period, when breasts tend to be less swollen and tender.

Blood Tests

At 35, I recommend a simple haemogram with haemoglobin, Vitamin-B12 with Vitamin-D3, a blood sugar fasting test if you have a family history of diabetes in and a serum cholesterol test as well.

Why do you need it? Indian women are highly prone to iron deficiency anaemia and Hb test will help detect that. Most vegetarians may display B12 deficiency while D3 deficiency seems to be on the rise. Since Vitamin-D3 is needed for calcium absorption, it is good to keep a tab on it.

Lifestyle diseases like diabetes and elevated lipid levels are risk factors for cardiac disease. For people with history of such diseases in the family, it is good to get these tests done in your early thirties.

Blood Sugar

If you look at any test you do in a laboratory, there will be your value, next to which will be the range of normal values. the body is in a constant state of work, metabolising, assimilating and excreting nutrients and toxins respectively.

Everyone's blood has sugar molecules to provide energy and to aid in various metabolic processes. When we eat, sugar values rise, giving us more energy. So if we check the sugar even after the body has had no food eight to ten hours, there will still be some sugar in the blood. This is called the fasting blood sugar lever and is measured in milligrams (mg) per decilitre (dl). A normal fasting blood glucose reading is below 100 mg/dl. If your results come in between 100 and 125 mg/dl, you are considered pre-diabetic and you should take this as a wake-up call. Losing a few pounds, about seven per cent of your total body weight, can put you back in the safe zone. If your FPG is 126 mg/dl or above, you are likely to have diabetes, a chronic, usually irreversible condition with lifelong repercussions. Requiring lifestyle modifications.

A more accurate screening for diabetes is the haemoglobin A1C test. Whereas a fasting blood test is like a snapshot, the A1C examines a protein in the blood that changes in the presence of too much blood sugar, indicating a blood glucose level over three to four month period. An A1C at 5.6 per cent, that means the percentage of sugar in your blood, is normal; a pre-diabetic range is between 5.7 and 6.4 per cent. Anything over that indicates diabetes.

Lipid Profile and Cholesterol

A lipid profile tests the following: S. cholesterol, S. triglycerides and some lipo proteins like LDL, HDL and VLDL. Keep in mind that cholesterol isn't a disease or condition; it's a factor that can indicate your risk of developing heart disease. What you should aim for is not just keeping your LDL low—100 mg/dl is optimal, but inching your HDL higher. The optimal measure here is over 60mg/dl, according to American Heart Association (AHA) standards. The total number to aim for is 200 mg/dl or less; a reading of over 240 is considered high.

The measure of triglycerides, the most common type of fat in your body, is a key number—inching over 150 mg/dl should send a red signal because a high triglyceride level combined with low HDL or high LDL may speed up atherosclerosis, the build-up of fatty deposits in artery walls, increasing your risk of a heart attack.

You should repeat this test every five years, more often if you have a family history of heart disease, or if you smoke or are overweight/obese.

Thyroid Check

Don't assume it's the kids or the boss or the husband or the maid if you're feeling chronically rundown. Thyroid issues, while they usually crop up later in life, are sometimes triggered by having a baby, and can wreak havoc on your energy levels.

The gold-standard thyroid test is a blood screening for TSH, or thyroid stimulating hormone, which detects hyperthyroidism, an overactive thyroid, causing insomnia and weight loss; or hypothyroidism, an underactive thyroid, causing sluggishness and weight gain. Get checked if you have symptoms such as unexplained changes in mood, weight gain/loss, irregular sleeping habits or cholesterol levels.

Blood Pressure

You must have had that familiar BP check every time you go to a doctor's office, but now's the time to start paying closer attention to it, especially if you have any risk for heart disease or stroke—a strong family history, being overweight or if you smoke.

Numbers to worry about: a systolic, or top reading between 120 and 139 and a diastolic, or bottom reading between 80 and 89 puts you in a pre-hypertensive state. Hypertension—high blood pressure—is defined as 140/90 or higher.

How often do you need it? Testing once a year is sufficient.

Fitness in Your 40s

40 today is definitely not what it meant for our mothers. For one thing, many of us in this decade still have young children around, not to mention feeling younger from eating well and exercising regularly. And really, how many of our moms were running marathons or doing ninety minutes of zumba at this age?

But the number is still meaningful when it comes to your health. At age forty and beyond, a woman's risk of developing conditions such as high blood pressure, heart disease, osteoporosis, diabetes and arthritis increase, and hence annual check-ups are a must! But there's still plenty of good news: many of these diseases can be skirted or slowed if you make smart, healthy lifestyle choices.

And this is where our mothers scored. They cooked more at home, ate out less and generally spent more time naturally looking after themselves, all of which we definitely need to emulate.

Healthy habits in place, this is the decade to take a hard look at family history. Take breast cancer for example: If you have a parent or a sibling who had the disease, you should get yourself tested ten years before the age when the disease was detected in your relative. This is the general rule of the thumb. And in addition to all the tests mentioned in your 30s, these are the other tests you must do.

Mammogram

Though there are conflicting recommendations, the general consensus is that mammograms with ultrasound are a good screening tool for detecting early stages of breast cancer; early detection can really make a world of difference. Mammograms are basically X-rays. There are film (traditional) and digital mammograms. Both are effective for spotting tumours, but research shows that digital mammography is significantly better for women who are younger than age 50 or have very dense breasts.

How often should one do it? Once a year.

Tip: Schedule mammos about two weeks after your period, when the breasts are less tender. Some women have denser breast tissues, especially when they are younger. So watch out for false positives.

Eye Examination

So you seem to be holding your mobile phone a little farther away from your face. What you have is a condition called presbyopia, a shortening of focus that's also known as short arm syndrome.

If you already wear glasses, see your ophthalmologist to discuss whether you should have separate reading glasses or a bifocal one. Those who have never seen an eye doctor should make an appointment for a comprehensive test that can pick up early signs of age-related problems such as cataract, glaucoma, diabetic retinopathy, age-related macular degeneration that may be lurking around without any manifested symptoms.

The exam will also include an eye pressure test, pupil dilation so the doctor can look at your retina and optic nerve, and a test of visual acuity, or reading letters on an eye chart.

How often should one do these tests? At least once every couple of years.

Dental Screening

Why do you need it? To rule out oral cancer and to combat gum disease and tooth decay.

When and how often? Twice a year teeth cleanings and check-ups should begin six months after your baby teeth appear, and continue for life. If you're pregnant or taking contraceptives, you may be more prone to gum inflammation. Smokers and women who have more than a drink or two a day are at a greater risk of gum disease and oral cancers.

I have seen many women in their thirties, in my practice who have never visited a dentist. Their usual explanation is that they do not have any teeth problems! Many of them take their children for braces etc, but never make an appointment for themselves. Hence, I am making a point here to tell you to visit a dentist at least once or twice a year for just a check up and to do some prevention as recommended.

A dentist will take a close look at all your teeth, your tongue, the soft and hard tissues of your mouth and neck and the area around your jaw to determine if there are any unusual changes in tissue. If you have gum disease, he or she may recommend that you return for cleanings more than twice a year. If have plaque and tartar, get your teeth scraped both above and below the gum line. If you have abnormal tissue growths, your dentist may ask you to do a biopsy.

50: The New 40

Thanks to increased awareness about nutrition and exercise, many women are taking care of themselves and remaining vibrant throughout this decade. But after menopause, women lose some of the protection that oestrogen had offered during their childbearing years, thereby increasing the risk of health problems such as osteoporosis and heart disease.

And the latter is actually the big one. It is a shocking fact that more women die of heart disease than they do of breast cancer. Annual tests are a must, and that should include blood pressure checks thrice a year and cholesterol test once a year. Keeping your weight under control is especially important: declining oestrogen levels cause fat storage to shift from the hips to the waist, and increased abdominal fat raises your risk of diabetes and heart disease.

This is also the decade to do a complete cardiovascular examination including an ECG, an echocardiogram and a stress test, all as advised by and under the supervision of a cardiologist. Occasionally, a 24 hour ECG monitoring called Holter monitoring may be needed. This is especially required for those with risk factors like high blood pressure, diabetes or high cholesterol, or those with a family history of cardiovascular illness. These tests can detect early signs and stem the damage right at the root itself.

Bone Scan

Most women do not need a bone scan till well into their 60s. However, if you are a smoker or have been on steroid-based medications for a large part of your life, you may want to do a bone scan in your 50s, to detect early osteoporosis.

Colonoscopy

It is necessary to do a Faecal Occult Blood Test (FOBT) for blood in your stool to detect any early sign of colon rectal cancer. If the doctor then recommends a colonoscopy, one must go ahead and do it as colon cancer, caught in time, can have very good treatment outcomes.

An ounce of prevention is really worth a pound of cure. All these tests cover the basic, common conditions that every woman must get tested for. Over and above these, there are specialized tests such as a hormone profile, X-rays of lungs, ultrasound of abdomen and pelvis which the doctor may recommend depending on specific symptoms that you display. These tests, done on time, will ensure that you maintain significantly good health in every decade of your life.

TESTS IN YOUR 30s

First complete physical

Pap Smear

Blood work

- ❑ Haemoglobin
- ❑ Cholesterol
- ❑ Sugar
- ❑ Thyroid function
- ❑ Liver and kidney function
- ❑ Vitamin-B12, D3

TESTS IN YOUR 40s

Mammogram

Lipid profile

Eye examination

Gynaecological exam

Cardiac check

TESTS IN YOUR 50s

Complete Cardiac Check-up

- ❑ ECG
- ❑ Echo
- ❑ X-ray
- ❑ Stress test
- ❑ Holter
- ❑ Bone scan
- ❑ Stool: Occult blood
- ❑ Colonoscopy

3

The JB Self-Test

Jelly Belly is, to me, less physical and more a metaphor of the average woman's attitude to health. The most visible physical attribute that one often spots in otherwise slim women is their tendency to have a protruding belly. This is a sign of poor health.

There could be a number of other tiny signs that may indicate that your health is poor—small, niggling things that you have been postponing paying attention to. So how do you know you ought to be taking greater care of yourself? Do the JB Test.

The JB Test

- ❑ Would you say your health is worse this year than it was in the last one?
- ❑ Do you feel your health is worse than that of the women around you?
- ❑ Do you feel tired by 7 p.m. on most days?
- ❑ Do you get a twinge in your neck, back or heel at least once a week?

- ❑ In the last six months, have you made a resolve to go on a diet more than thrice but not got around to it?
- ❑ Do you get a physical examination done at least once a year?
- ❑ Have your periods changed its pattern in the last one year?
- ❑ Do you find yourself arguing more than you ever used to, or throwing your hands up in frustration?
- ❑ Do you have a family history of diabetes or high blood pressure in either parents or siblings?
- ❑ Do you constantly look at yourself in the mirror and think you look fat, your tummy looks big, your skin is terrible, your hair lacks volume or lustre?
- ❑ Do you get out of breath when you walk up two flights of stairs?
- ❑ Have you had more than one bout of ill-health like fever, diarrhoea, burning urine or severe head or back ache which has incapacitated you in the last one year?

If you have answered yes to more than five of these questions, then you definitely are in a JB state of health and need to focus on gaining it back. If you have answered yes to less than five of these, congratulations, you are in good shape. But read on to see how you can maintain this state of wonderful health and well-being and make it an indelible part of your life.

4

Jelly Belly

It's been described by various names: middle-aged spread, dumbbell roll, muffin top and the more prosaic tummy fat. But to me, the most evocative symbol of unwanted weight gain is the jelly belly. I was in conversation with my friend Dr Sarita Subramanian which went like this, imagine you have just come back home from a nice dinner with friends and are getting ready for bed. You unsnap the button of your stretch jeans, roll down the zipper and out pops your belly, all aquiver. This is jelly belly which afflicts a lot of us in our late 20s, 30s and 40s, not only us chubby ones but sometimes even those of us who are slim or skinny.

Jelly bellies are the most obvious indications of problematic and unwanted fat depositions in one's body. What makes their appearance worse is the fact that they are sometimes generously peppered with stretch marks. Very often, they have an overhang where tonelessly the fat flaps and flops over the lower abdomen and balloons up when you lie down.

The other area where fat deposits is the famous bobbly double chin. But the difference is that whereas the cause of double chins are almost always genetic and their effect is purely aesthetic, jelly bellies can have serious health implications and hence warrant a closer look.

Why Does One Get a Jelly Belly?

There are many reasons for it. The most obvious ones are, of course, eating the wrong type of food coupled with a total lack of exercise.

Jelly belly does not begin in the mid-30s, but becomes most evident at this age. Of course, if you are pregnant, you will have a growing big belly, but that is a reason for joy, not a cause for concern and this section does not apply to you. By 30 your primary female hormone production—oestrogen and progesterone—begin to slow down promoting fat deposition in certain localized areas like the belly, chin and upper arms. Also there is an imbalance between the two hormones. This is because fat cells produce oestrogen which now your body craves. This is because fat cells contain an enzyme called aromatase, an enzyme required for biosynthesis of oestrogen.

The trouble with hormonal belly fat is that it's not limited to the extra layer of padding located just below the skin that you can pinch up (subcutaneous fat). It also includes visceral fat—which lies deep inside your abdomen, surrounding your internal organs. Whereas subcutaneous fat poses cosmetic concerns, visceral fat is associated with far more dangerous health consequences. That's because an excessive amount of visceral fat produces hormones that can raise blood pressure, negatively alter good and bad cholesterol levels. Good cholesterol is what helps in protecting the heart while bad cholesterol can form plaques in our blood vessels slowing down blood flow. Excessive fat also impairs the body's ability to use insulin (insulin resistance). For any activity done, the higher your fat and lower the muscle, the less calories you will burn. All of this can increase the risk of serious health problems including cardiovascular disease, stroke, Type-2 diabetes, and even make us more susceptible to some kinds of cancers like breast and colon rectal.

Let's look closely at the different hormones that play a role in having a jelly belly.

Oestrogen: Oestrogen is the female sex hormone that is responsible for causing monthly ovulation. During and following ovulation, oestrogen levels start declining and continue to decline up to menopause when they cause your ovaries to stop ovulating. More relevantly for us here, oestrogen plays a big role in fat gain. As the ovaries produce less oestrogen, the body looks for other places to grab oestrogen from. Fat cells in the body can produce oestrogen, so your body works harder to convert calories into fat to increase oestrogen levels. Unfortunately, fat cells don't burn calories the way muscle cells do, which causes the unwanted pounds.

Progesterone: During ovulation and thereafter, progesterone levels will also decrease. Like oestrogen, lower levels of this hormone can be responsible for weight gain, or at least the appearance of it. Water retention and bloating are caused by decreased progesterone levels. Though this doesn't actually result in permanent weight gain, your clothes will probably feel a bit tighter and you may feel a bit heavier adding to the overall feeling of being overweight.

Androgens: These hormones, or the male hormones, are responsible for sending your newly added weight directly to the middle of your body. It could signify the beginnings of menopause. An increase in androgens, which typically can happen around menopause, will exhibit other signs like increasing facial hair.

Other than hormonal imbalances, once you touch forty, you could develop a condition called insulin resistance. Insulin is a hormone produced in our bodies which helps in digestion by breaking down the carbohydrates we eat into digestible sugars, most importantly, glucose. Insulin is a hormone made by the pancreas. It helps cells absorb glucose (sugar) from the blood to use as energy. Your body digests foods that contain carbohydrates and releases them as glucose into your blood. Insulin, which is released when you eat, helps the body maintain a healthy level of circulating glucose by allowing glucose from the blood to go into the cells. This lowers blood sugar, and the cells use the glucose for energy.

Insulin resistance is a condition in which the body produces insulin but does not use it properly. Some people may begin to have problems using insulin correctly. This is referred to as insulin resistance. With insulin resistance, your pancreas produces insulin, but your cells aren't using it as well as they should. When insulin is not working the way it should, your cells don't absorb glucose properly, which leads to a buildup of sugar in your blood. If your blood glucose levels are higher than normal but aren't high enough to be considered Type-2 diabetes, you are said to have prediabetes.

When people are insulin resistant, their muscle, fat and liver cells do not respond properly to insulin. As a result, their bodies need more insulin to help the glucose enter the cells. The pancreas tries to keep up with this increased demand for insulin by producing more. Eventually, the pancreas fails to keep up with the body's need for insulin. Excess glucose builds up in the bloodstream, setting the stage for diabetes. Many people with insulin resistance have high levels of both glucose and insulin circulating in their blood at the same time. Hence, insulin resistance is also considered a pre-diabetic syndrome, and deposition of belly fat could be one of the early visible signs of insulin resistance, although the belly itself does not influence production of insulin. Abdominal fat cells can disrupt the normal balance and functioning of hormones such as leptin and adiponectin, which are thought to play a role in your body's response to insulin, according to Harvard University Medical School. Since insulin resistance has no symptoms but predisposes to diabetes, increased abdominal fat is a warning signal that helps us identify at risk people for the same.

Another condition which has a jelly belly as an integral component is the much debated metabolic syndrome. This is a combination of five factors: abdominal fat (waist measurement greater than 35 inches), increased cholesterol or taking cholesterol medication, high blood pressure or on blood pressure medication and high blood sugar or on blood sugar medication. Metabolic syndrome itself is considered to indicate hormonal imbalance, an increase in oestrogen and cholesterol, and an increase in androgens in women—all of which predispose a woman to deposit fat on the belly, or become apple shaped.

Deficiency of the thyroxin hormone produced by the

thyroid gland could be yet another reason why women tend to gain weight around their waists. It is accompanied by lethargy, a feeling of tiredness and an inability to tolerate cold temperatures. This can be easily detected by a physician with a simple blood test.

If one were to look at the causes mentioned above, it will be obvious that they are all interlinked. The good news is that remedial measures that help in tackling one of them can also control some of the other causal factors.

Causes of Jelly Belly

- Heredity
- Improper diet
- Lack of exercise
- Insulin resistance
- Hormonal imbalance
- Hypothyroidism
- Metabolic syndrome

Measure It Up

Although some of the causal factors may require a more detailed testing as recommended by doctors, diagnosing that you have a jelly belly is really not that tough. All you have to do is measure your waist circumference in the proper way. All you need is to stand in front of a mirror and do the following:

- Place a tape above your hipbone which is around your bare stomach.
- Pull the tape until it fits snugly around you without being tight or pinching your skin.

- Check in the mirror that the tape measure is at the same level all around.
- Relax, breathe out and measure your waist.
- Do not breathe in or suck in your stomach.

Although the definition for metabolic syndrome is 35 inches, I tell all my patients to consider 33 inches as their personal warning to sit up and take note. Jelly Belly is on its way in!

If you do fall in this category, I would recommend a visit to your physician. Any test that you may require to diagnose insulin resistance, hypothyroidism, etc., can be determined by your physician by simple blood tests after doing a clinical examination.

Waist Management

You can tone abdominal muscles with crunches or other targeted abdominal exercises, but these exercises won't get rid of belly fat. Fortunately, however, deep tummy fat responds to the same diet and exercise strategies that can help you shed excess pounds and lower your total body fat. To fight back the bulge, stick to a simple three point programme: DIP into your jelly to take it off!

- *Diet:* Choose to eat plant-based foods, such as fruits, vegetables and whole grains, and choose lean sources of protein and low-fat dairy products. Limit bad fats found in red meat and high-fat dairy products, such as cheese and butter. Include in moderation the good fats found in fish, nuts and certain vegetable oils like olive and sunflower oils.

- *Include and increase physical activity*: For most healthy adults moderate aerobic activity, such as brisk walking, for at least 150 minutes a week, or vigorous aerobic activity, such as jogging, for at least 75 minutes a week, is recommended to burn fat. In addition, as I mentioned before in an earlier chapter, strength training exercises like weights, pilates or yoga are recommended at least twice a week. If you want to lose weight or meet specific fitness goals, you may need to exercise more.
- *Portion Control*: Whatever you may eat including the healthy foods, limit your portion size. Count the number of servings, start by reducing them by 25 per cent, and build up to halving it. Eat small, more frequent meals during the day rather than three big meals.

Can Pills Help?

Pills can only help you if you have an identified underlying cause. For instance, if you have hypothyroidism, thyroxin can be prescribed, there are drugs for insulin resistance, and metabolic syndrome can be treated with anti-cholesterol drugs. All these have to be taken under medical supervision only and monitored for side effects. Again, pills can only improve the results you obtain from DIP, not serve as a substitute for it!

Additional DIP Tips from JB Pals

Over the years, I have come across several patients and friends who have battled their jelly bellies successfully. I am sharing some of their strategies with you.

DIP Tips

- ❏ Drink plenty of water—helps tremendously
- ❏ Drink unsweetened green tea
- ❏ Eat your dinner early, preferably by 7 p.m.
- ❏ Always have a large bowl of soup as your first course for dinner
- ❏ Eat an omelette made of egg whites or a vegetarian omelette with chick pea flour at least thrice a week
- ❏ When you crave a particular food like chocolate, eat a piece of it immediately. Your craving will stop
- ❏ Eat oats and brown rice regularly
- ❏ Do abs exercises to tone the belly muscles
- ❏ Do not go on crash/fad diets—they all rebound
- ❏ Eat very light, grain-free food once a week—it is super effective
- ❏ We all plateau, so do not lose heart, and just persist with it
- ❏ Do not reward yourself for weight loss with food; shop for a tighter dress instead
- ❏ Sleep well: it is still the best kept slimness secret
- ❏ Be happy and reduce stress! It will speed up your slimming

Most importantly, do remember, you are not alone. A lot of us are afflicted by the same issues, so hang in there and stick to your diet and exercise regimen, compare notes with friends and peers, and soon, the jelly will roll away for sure!

TO SUMMARIZE

What is it? A floppy lower tummy without tone

Who gets it? Anyone, common in multi-pregnancy and hormonally afflicted women

Diagnosis: Measuring the waist, more than 35 inches

Underlying causes: Hormones, insulin resistance, metabolic syndrome

Treatment: DIP approach

- ❑ Diet
- ❑ Include Exercise
- ❑ Portion control

5

The Heart Truth

Whenever I speak to any of my patients or friends about heart disease, the usual response is: 'Isn't that something women are protected against? Why do I have to worry?'

Well, the hard truth is that a lot of women suffer from and die of heart or cardiovascular irregularities. While it is true that oestrogen does provide a certain protective effect, our lifestyles combined with modern stress levels make us particularly vulnerable to heart diseases.

Why is there a rising concern about women and heart health?

For a long time, it was believed that women are more protected from heart disease because of their hormones. However it has become increasingly evident that this is no longer true in its entirety. Rising stress levels, due to changing roles for women, juggling multiple commitments and increasing lifestyle risks have unfortunately changed this and has placed women at high risk for increasingly poor heart health.

In the Global context, WHO pegs that 8.4 million women

die of heart disease, out of which a whopping 34 per cent are from India. A recent study done in 2015 by Saffola Life Foundation revealed that three out of five women in India are at risk for heart disease. Further, doctors surveyed as part of the visualising extent of heart disease in women study overwhelmingly (81 per cent) felt that women are neglectful of their own health and are less proactive than men in seeking early tests and help to protect their hearts. This definitely indicates the magnitude of the problem and the need to protect your heart by appropriate remedial measures.

Coronary heart disease, often simply called heart disease, occurs when the arteries that supply blood to the heart muscle become hardened and narrowed due to a build-up of plaque on the arteries' inner walls. Plaque is the accumulation of fat, cholesterol and other substances. As plaque continues to build up in the arteries, blood flow to the heart gets reduced.

Heart disease can lead to a heart attack. A heart attack happens when an artery becomes totally blocked with plaque, preventing vital oxygen and nutrients from reaching the heart. A heart attack can cause permanent damage to the heart muscle.

Heart disease is one of the several cardiovascular diseases, which are diseases of the heart and blood vessel system. Other cardiovascular diseases include stroke, high blood pressure and rheumatic heart disease.

A lot of people think heart disease can be 'cured' with surgery. This is a myth. Heart disease is a lifelong condition—once you get it, you'll always have it. It is true that procedures such as bypass surgery and angioplasty can help blood and oxygen flow to the heart more easily. But the arteries remain damaged, which means you are more likely to have a heart attack.

What's more, the condition of your blood vessels will steadily worsen unless you make changes in your daily habits.

Prevention of disease begins with first knowing your susceptibility and risk factors that may make you prone to heart disease. Some risk factors are out of your control—that include age and family history. If a female member of your family, your mother or sibling, has got a heart disease before 60, chances are that you are vulnerable too. The average age that women are most susceptible seems to be 53 (50-55), though women with no risk factors may not be susceptible till in their 60s.

Regardless of these statistics, prevention of heart disease must start as early as in your mid-30s. Let us take a look at some of the risk factors that can be mitigated by preventive interventions.

It must be understood that having even one of the risk factors mentioned below increases your risk two-fold. Having two of them quadruples it, and more than two risk factors increases your risk multiple times. Hence, understanding them and making suitable interventions are extremely crucial.

Risk factors for heart disease: They can be summed up by an acronym: **BP LESS**

- A BMI of over 25
- High blood pressure
- Lipid profile
- Lack of exercise
- High blood sugar
- Smoking and stress

BMI stands for body mass index and is the most commonly used weight indicator to assess risk. It is calculated in the following way:

Weight in kilograms divided by the square of your height in metres.

So if your weight is 65 kg and your height is 5 ft 4 inches, convert 5 ft to inches by multiplying by 12, so 60 inches.

Add 4 inches so the total is 64 inches.

Multiply this by 2.54 to get your height in centimetre.

So your height in cms is 162.56 cms.

This in metre is 1.6256 meter.

The square of this is 2.64257536

So your BMI is 65/2.64257536 = 24.6

A BMI of 18.5 to 24.9 indicates a normal weight.

A person with a BMI from 25-29.9 is overweight, while someone with a BMI of 30 or higher is obese.

Those in the 'overweight' or 'obese' categories have a higher risk of heart disease.

So what should you do?

- ❑ If you are obese, you should lose weight.
- ❑ If you are overweight, have a waist measurement of more than 35 inches, *and* have two or more other risk factors, you should lose weight.
- ❑ If you are overweight, but do not have a high waist measurement and have fewer than two other risk factors, you should avoid further weight gain.

A small weight loss of just five to ten per cent of your current weight will help lower your risk of heart disease and other serious medical disorders. The best way to shed the kilos is to do so gradually, by getting more physical activity and following a heart healthy eating plan that is lower in calories and fat. (High-fat foods contain more calories than the same amount of other foods. But be careful—'low fat' doesn't always mean low in calories. Sometimes extra sugars are added to low-fat desserts, for example.)

High Blood Sugar: Diabetes Mellitus

Diabetes is a serious medical condition that must be taken seriously. In Type-2 diabetes, the pancreas produces insulin, but the body cannot use it properly and gradually loses the ability to produce it. Type-2 diabetes is a serious disease. In addition to increasing the risk of heart ailments, it is a leading cause of kidney failure, eye and feet problems in adults. Diabetes can also lead to nerve damage and loss of immunity in fighting infection.

The risk of Type-2 diabetes rises after the age of 45. You are more likely to develop it if you are overweight, especially if you have extra kilos around the waist. Other risk factors include physical inactivity and a family history of diabetes. India is today the diabetes capital of the world indicating underlying genetic and lifestyle causes.

Women who have had diabetes during pregnancy (gestational diabetes) or have given birth to a baby weighing more than nine pounds are more likely to develop Type-2 diabetes later on in life. Symptoms of diabetes include fatigue, nausea, frequent urination, unusual thirst, weight loss, blurred vision, frequent infections and slow healing of sores. But sometimes there are no symptoms. Even if you have no symptoms of diabetes, if you are overweight and have any of the risk factors, you must get tested for it. It is recommended that you fast and do the post-prandial blood sugar test as well as the HBA1C test.

If you have diabetes, controlling your blood glucose (blood sugar) levels will help to prevent complications. Because diabetes is so strongly linked with heart disease, managing diabetes must include keeping other risk factors like blood pressure and cholesterol under control as well. Not smoking, being physically active, and taking aspirin daily (if your doctor recommends it) also are important ways to prevent heart disease if you have diabetes.

Some people do not yet have diabetes but are at high risk for developing the disease. They have a condition known as 'prediabetes', in which blood glucose levels are higher than normal but not yet in the diabetic range. But new research shows that many people with prediabetes can prevent or delay the development of diabetes by making modest changes in their diet and level of physical activity.

Cholesterol/Lipid Profile

High blood cholesterol is another major risk factor for developing heart disease. The higher your blood cholesterol level, the greater your risk of a heart attack. So women should make a serious effort to keep their cholesterol at healthy levels. If you already have a heart disease, it is particularly important to lower an elevated blood cholesterol level to reduce risk of a heart attack. Women with diabetes are at an especially high risk.

Although young women tend to have lower cholesterol levels than young men, between the ages of 45 and 55, women's levels begin to rise surpassing men's. After 55, this 'cholesterol gap' between women and men becomes still wider. Although women's overall risk of heart disease at older ages continues to be somewhat lower than that of men, the higher a woman's blood cholesterol level, the greater her chances of developing a heart disease.

The body needs cholesterol to function normally. However, the body produces all the cholesterol it needs. Over a period of years, extra cholesterol and fat circulating in the blood build up in the walls of the arteries that supply blood to the heart. This build-up, called plaque, makes the arteries narrower and narrower. As a result, less blood reaches the heart. Blood carries oxygen. If not enough oxygen-rich blood can reach your heart, you may suffer chest pain. If the blood supply to a portion of the heart is completely cut off, the result is a heart attack.

Cholesterol travels in the blood in packages or parcels called lipoproteins. LDL carries most of the cholesterol in the blood. Cholesterol in LDL is often called 'bad' cholesterol, because too much LDL in the blood can lead to cholesterol build up and blockage in the arteries.

Another type of cholesterol is HDL, also known as 'good' cholesterol. That's because HDL helps remove cholesterol from the body, preventing it from building up in the arteries.

High blood cholesterol itself does not cause symptoms, so if your cholesterol level is high, you may not be aware of it. That's why it's important to get your cholesterol levels checked regularly. Starting from the age of 20, all women should have their cholesterol levels checked by means of a blood test called a 'fasting lipoprotein profile.'

Total cholesterol is a measure of the cholesterol in all of your lipoproteins, including the 'bad' cholesterol in LDL and the 'good' cholesterol in HDL. An LDL level below 100 mg/dl* is considered 'optimal,' or ideal. However, not every woman needs to aim for so low a level. Suffice to know, the higher your LDL number, the higher your risk of heart disease. Knowing your LDL number is especially important because it will determine the kind of treatment you may need.

Your HDL number is diametrically opposite. The lower your HDL level, the higher your heart disease risk. Your lipoprotein profile test will also measure levels of triglycerides, another fatty substance in the blood. This is a measure of the fat in your body, which then indicates the risk of the fat getting deposited in your arteries. Triglycerides are one major type of fat found in the blood and in food.

Triglycerides are produced in the liver. When you drink alcohol or take in more calories than your body needs, your liver produces more triglycerides. Triglyceride levels that are borderline high (150–199 mg/dl) or high (200–499 mg/dl) are signals of an increased risk of heart disease. To reduce blood triglyceride levels, it is important to control your weight, get more physical activity, quit smoking, and avoid alcohol. You should also follow an eating plan that is not too high in carbohydrates (less than 60 per cent of calories) and is low in saturated fat, trans fat and cholesterol. Sometimes, medication is also needed.

The Numbers

Blood Cholesterol Levels and Heart Disease Risk

- Total Cholesterol Level—Less than 200 mg/dl: Ideal
- 200–239 mg/dl: Borderline high
- 240 mg/dl and above: High

LDL Cholesterol Level—Less than 100 mg/dl: Ideal

- 100–129 mg/dl: Near ideal
- 130–159 mg/dl: Borderline high
- 160–189 mg/dl: High
- 190 mg/dl upwards: Very high

HDL Cholesterol—Less than 40 mg/dl: Risk High

Lowering Your Risk

The aim of all cholesterol control focuses primarily on lowering your LDL levels. There are two main ways to do that:

- Lifestyle changes alone
- Medication combined with lifestyle changes.

Depending on your risk, motivation and desire to make those changes and your doctor's approach, you must make a choice about which of the two will work for you.

Lifestyle Changes

One important treatment approach is called the TLC Programme, as recommended by the American Cardiology

Association Guidelines. TLC stands for 'Therapeutic Lifestyle Changes,' a three-part treatment that uses diet, physical activity and weight management. Maintaining a healthy weight and getting regular physical activity are especially important for women who have metabolic syndrome as discussed in chapter one.

If your LDL level stays too high even after making lifestyle changes, you may need to take medicine. If you need medication, be sure to use it along with the TLC approach. This will keep the dose of medicine as low as possible and lower your risk in other ways as well. You will also need to control all your other heart disease risk factors, including high blood pressure, diabetes and smoking.

High Blood Pressure

High blood pressure, also known as hypertension, is another major risk factor for heart disease, as well as for kidney disease and congestive heart failure. High blood pressure is also the most important risk factor for stroke.

Major contributors to high blood pressure are a family history of the disease, excess weight, and eating a diet high in sodium. The older you are, the higher the risk. And women are more likely than men to develop high blood pressure.

High blood pressure is often called the 'silent killer,' because it usually doesn't cause any easily observable symptoms. As a result, many people pay little attention to their blood pressure until they become seriously ill. The good news is that you can take action to control or prevent high blood pressure, and thereby avoid many life-threatening disorders.

What Is Blood Pressure?

Blood pressure is the amount of force exerted by the blood against the walls of the arteries. Everyone has to have some blood pressure so that blood can get to all of the body's organs. Usually, blood pressure is expressed as two numbers, such as 120/80, and is measured in millimetres of mercury (mmHg).

The first number is the systolic blood pressure, the amount of force used when the heart beats. The second number, or diastolic blood pressure, is the pressure that exists in the arteries (the pipes for oxygenated blood) between heartbeats.

Because blood pressure changes often, your doctor will and should check it on several different days before deciding whether your blood pressure is too high.

High blood pressure can be controlled in two ways: by changing your lifestyle and by taking medication.

So What Is High Blood Pressure?

Your blood pressure is determined by the higher number of either your systolic or your diastolic measurement. For example, if your systolic number is 116 mmHg but your diastolic number is 96 mmHg, you have diastolic hypertension.

Systolic and Diastolic

Normal: Less than 120 mmHg/Less than 80 mmHg

Prehypertension: 120–139 mmHg/80–89 mmHg

Hypertension: 140 mmHg or higher/90 mmHg or higher

If your blood pressure is not too high, you may be able to control it entirely by losing weight if you are overweight, getting regular physical activity, cutting down on alcohol, and changing your eating habits. Nutritional approach is very important as is cutting down on salt.

If after a fair trial of three months, it continues to stay high, you must see your doctor again and consider starting medication. However, the lifestyle changes must continue.

Smoking

The last risk factor in the context of cardiac disease is smoking. Smoking is one of the leading causes of preventable death and disease. Women who smoke are two to six times more likely to suffer a heart attack than non-smoking women, and the risk increases with the number of cigarettes inhaled each day. Smoking can also shorten a healthy life, because smokers are likely to suffer a heart attack or other major heart problem at least ten years sooner than non-smokers. Smoking also raises the risk of stroke.

But heart disease and stroke are not the only health risks for women who smoke. Smoking greatly increases the chances that a woman will develop lung cancer. In fact, the lung cancer death rate for women is now higher than the death rate for breast cancer. Cigarette smoking also causes many other types of cancer, including cancers of the mouth, urinary tract, kidney and cervix. Smoking also causes most cases of chronic obstructive lung disease, which includes bronchitis and emphysema. If you smoke indoors, the 'second-hand smoke' from your cigarettes can cause heart disease, lung cancer and other serious health problems in the non-smokers around you. Second-hand smoke is especially harmful for infants and young children, causing breathing problems, ear infections, asthma attacks and sudden infant death syndrome (SIDS).

There is simply no safe way to smoke. Low-tar and low-nicotine cigarettes do not lessen the risks of heart disease or other smoking-related diseases. The only safe and healthful course is not to smoke at all.

Having looked at the top risk factors for heart disease, we can see that three of them are completely related to lifestyle: namely weight, exercise and smoking. The other three are heavily influenced by lifestyle but since there are other factors which influence them too, it is important to look at them holistically and track them periodically. This tracking can be done by a simple ABC approach.

A is for the A1C test, which is short for haemoglobin A1C. This test measures your average blood glucose (blood sugar) over the previous three months. It lets you know if your blood glucose level is under control.

Get this test done at least twice a year. The number to aim for is below 6.5.

B is for blood pressure. The higher your blood pressure, the harder your heart has to work. Get your blood pressure measured at every doctor's visit. The numbers to aim for are at or below 130/80 mmHg.

C is for cholesterol. LDL, or 'bad' cholesterol, builds up and clogs your arteries. Get your LDL cholesterol tested at least once a year. The number to aim for is below 100 mg/dl.

Physical Activity and Exercise

Lack of physical activity and exercise raises your risk of heart disease more than you might think. It boosts your chances of developing heart-related problems even if you have no other risk factors. It also increases the likelihood that you will develop other heart disease risk factors such as high blood pressure, diabetes and obesity.

Yet most women aren't getting enough physical activity. Overall, older people are less likely to be active than younger individuals, and women tend to be less physically active than men. For women, physical inactivity also increases the risk of osteoporosis, which in turn may increase the risk of broken bones.

Fortunately, research shows that as little as 30 minutes of moderate activity on most, and preferably all, days of the week helps to protect your health. This level of activity can reduce your risk of heart disease as well as lower your chances of having a stroke, colon cancer, high blood pressure, diabetes, and other medical problems.

Examples of moderate activity are taking a brisk walk, dancing, light weightlifting, half hour of cardio at the gym, 30 minutes of zumba, one hour of yoga, and so on. If you prefer, you can divide your 30-minute activity into shorter periods of at least ten minutes each.

Tests That Can Help Protect Your Heart Health

Each of these tests will give you valuable information about your heart disease risk.

Lipoprotein Profile

What is it? A blood test that measures total cholesterol, HDL or 'good' cholesterol, LDL or 'bad' cholesterol, and triglycerides, another form of fat in the blood. The test is given after a 9 to12-hour fast.

Why should you do it? To find out if you have any of the following: high blood cholesterol (high total and LDL cholesterol), low HDL cholesterol, or high triglyceride levels. All affect your risk of heart disease.

When should you do it? All healthy adults should have their blood cholesterol levels checked at least once every five years. Depending on the results, your doctor may want to repeat the test more frequently.

Blood Pressure

What: A simple, painless test using an inflatable cuff on the arm.

Why: To find out if you have high blood pressure (also called hypertension) or prehypertension. Both are risk factors for heart disease.

When: At least every two years, or more often if you have high blood pressure or prehypertension.

Fasting Plasma Glucose

What: The preferred test for diagnosing diabetes. After you have fasted overnight, you should get a blood test done the following morning.

Why: To find out if you have diabetes or are likely to develop the disease. Fasting plasma glucose levels of more than 126 mg/dl on two tests on different days mean that you have diabetes. Levels between 100 and 125 mg/dl mean you have an increased risk of diabetes and may have prediabetes. Diabetes is an important risk factor for heart disease and other medical disorders.

When: At least every three years, beginning at age 45. If you have risk factors for diabetes, you should be tested at a younger age and more often.

Body Mass Index (BMI) and Waist Circumference

What: BMI is a measure of your weight in relation to your height. Waist circumference is a measure of the fat around your middle.

Why: To find out whether your body type raises your risk of heart disease. A BMI of 25 or higher means you are overweight. A BMI of 30 or higher means you are obese. Both overweight and obesity are risk factors for heart disease. For women, a waist measurement of more than 35 inches increases the risk of heart disease and other serious health conditions.

When: Every two years, or more often if your doctor recommends it.

Other Tests

There are several other tests that can determine whether you already have heart disease. Ask your doctor if you need other tests like a stress test; C-reactive protein, measuring homocysteine levels; an electrocardiogram (ECG) or another diagnostic test called Echocardiogram.

Be Hale and Hearty

Every single thing that we do to stay heart healthy and fit has to become a part of our lives. The lifestyle changes have to be gradual, lasting and permanent. There will be bad days and occasions when you slip up, but it is often said that if we practise anything diligently for 30 days, it becomes a part of our lives. Getting serious about heart health may seem like a huge project. But it doesn't have to be an overwhelming one.

Remember, nobody always eats the ideal diet or gets just the right amount of physical activity. Few smokers are able to swear off cigarettes without a slip or two along the way. The important thing is to follow a sensible, realistic plan that you will gradually grow into.

There are just a few things we need to do every day to keep ourselves healthy and heart safe. I'm going to list them below:

- ❑ Be physically active every day.
- ❑ Follow your doctor's advice about the type of physical activity but do it every day for at least 30 minutes.
- ❑ Eat less salt, saturated fat, trans fat and cholesterol-rich foods.
- ❑ Use cooking oil sparingly and use oils rich in MUFAs and PUFAs like olive, sunflower, safflower, rice bran and mustard oils.
- ❑ Eat more fibre. Choose fibre-rich whole grains like oats as part of your everyday diet.

- Ensure you include sufficient fruits, vegetables and beans of all kinds every single day.
- Stay at a healthy weight.
- If you smoke, stop completely. The benefits are tremendous.
- Take medicines as prescribed. And be regular with them.

TO SUMMARIZE

Heart Disease: Increasingly common in women, linked to family history, genetics and lifestyle

Risk factors for heart disease: BP LESS

- BMI
- Pressure (blood)
- Lipid Profile
- Exercise
- Sugar (blood)
- Smoking and Stress

Detection: Combination of self test, medical examinations, blood tests and cardiac work up

Prevention: Lifestyle changes to control risk factors

ABC approach:

- Prevention—Control diet, exercise regularly and get periodic tests done
- Control diabetes, high blood pressure and cholesterol

6

What's on Your Plate?

I have one honest confession to make here. I love food. I have a deep relationship with food, the cooking, the eating, the caring and sharing it denotes, the possibilities that it offers for both emotional and physical satisfaction. But I must confess food is often the bane of my life. I struggle to understand the complexities, the nutritional needs of my body, the foods that are good for me and the tastes that I crave.

There is so much information available on food. A lot of it is centred on diets, some of it around diet plans and a whole lot more on examination of various food groups and their nutritive value. But most women who speak to me are looking for something very simple. What does my body need for good health? What is good for me? What is bad? How do I make it tasty? How do I make the cooking easy? So, we are going to look at food from the perspective of finding answers to these simple questions.

I can also tell you from personal experience that changing the way we eat, in entirety, in our mid 30s and 40s is quite tough. Doubtless, there are women who do it, but the ones who sustain and stay on it are few and far in-between. We tend to 'become' good and try eating healthy for short, sometimes long, periods to achieve weight loss. But, especially for women in their 40s and above, what is needed is a sustainable approach to nutrition that can be maintained for the rest of their lives.

What Is a Calorie?

- A calorie is a measure of the energy used by the body and the energy that food supplies to the body. Carbohydrates, proteins, fats, alcohol all have calories. Your caloric needs are determined by your age, your size, how physically active you are, whether you are pregnant or breastfeeding, and other special conditions.
- Your caloric needs also depend on whether you want to lose or gain weight or keep your weight where it is.
- The quality of calories and where you get them from is as important as the total number for good nutrition.

Nutrition and Weight Loss

Last week, I was talking to one of my patients, Mrs Gupta, a lovely 42 year old woman, about her nutritional needs. The moment I asked her to describe her daily diet, she started bemoaning the fact that she is unable to lose weight. 'Doctor, I am on diets all the time. Yet, I do not seem to lose any weight. Just two days of bad eating and I seem to gain about two kilos. I have tried all the diets in the market. Even if I do lose some weight, it is invariably accompanied by hair loss, dull skin and an overall sense of fatigue. And I just did some tests, and my haemoglobin, calcium and Vitamin-D3 are all low and my cholesterol is high. What should I do?

Mrs Gupta is not isolated. I think most of us in our mid-30s upwards struggle with this. Nutrition becomes equivalent to weight loss and in a bid to lose weight quickly, we resort to starvation and fad diets, which tend to cause far more grave nutritional imbalances in our body. Coupled with the fact that we may be trying to conceive, dealing with menopause, etc., these nutritional imbalances tend to result into lifestyle diseases which then perpetuate the imbalances further. Inability to deal with not losing weight, in spite of denying ourselves food, sometimes causes depression which then leads into comfort eating. So, how do we free ourselves from this quagmire that seems inescapable?

The first thing to understand really is that every calorie is not the same. All foods, apart from their calorific value, have a different composition of nutrients. Some like carbohydrates, proteins and fats are called macronutrients, while others like minerals, vitamins, and anti-oxidants are called micronutrients. Food exchanges or different foods with the same calories give you a dizzying difference in micronutrients which actually make a world of difference in our ability to be healthy and lose weight. I'm going to give you a few examples:

- One serving of 28 g of potato chips which is 155 calories vs one bowl of oats which is 150 calories
- Two and a half cups of green beans vs 25 g of cheddar cheese, both of which are about 100 calories
- One small sweet baked potato vs half a tablespoon of butter, both of which are 55 calories

So calorie is not the only thing to look out for—it is equally important to count the nutritive value. So, how will you choose what to eat every day?

- *Focus on whole, plant-based foods.* Fill most of your plate with fruits and leafy green vegetables. Also include a variety of whole grains, beans and other legumes to keep you feeling full and energetic throughout the day. Try to find minimally processed or locally grown foods whenever possible and make these foods the mainstay of your diet.
- *Bone up on calcium.* Calcium is necessary for the growth and maintenance of strong teeth and bones, nerve signalling, muscle contraction and secretion of certain hormones and enzymes. Women are at a greater risk than men of developing osteoporosis, so it's important to get plenty of calcium to support your bone health. While dairy products are high in calcium, their animal fat and protein can accelerate bone loss. So consider plant-based sources of calcium like spinach, methi, beans, broccoli, kale, Brussels sprouts and collard greens. Other sources of calcium are fruits like orange, fig, grape; legumes like kidney bean and chickpea; nuts like almond, walnut and pistachio; and fish like salmon and mackerel.

Protein plays an important role in the biochemical, biophysical and physiological processes. Protein is required for all most all functions of the body as well as the structural integrity of cells. Protein regulates the gene, the basic building block of life, and is present in different enzymes and hormones. Enzymes are the catalysts that enable different chemical activities in the body while hormones are those complex substances that control and stimulate organs like the pituitary, thyroid, ovaries etc. Eating the right type of protein is important because although protein is an essential part of any healthy diet, eating too much animal-based protein—(such as the levels recommended in many low-carb, high-protein diets)—is particularly dangerous for women. It can cause calcium loss and lead to a decrease in bone density and osteoporosis.

Include iron in your diet. Iron is required for the production of red blood cells (a process known as haematopoiesis) but it's also a part of haemoglobin which is the red pigment of the red blood cells) Haemoglobin is the substance in blood which binds to the oxygen and facilitates its transport from the lungs to all cells throughout the body for their proper functioning.

Once the oxygen is delivered the iron (as part of haemoglobin), then binds to the carbon dioxide which is then transported back to the lung from where it gets exhaled. So essentially, it is the backbone of all life processes as it delivers oxygen and excretes carbon dioxide from all living cells.

Some sources of iron would be vegetables like spinach, methi and amaranth; pulses like soybeans and kidney beans; whole grains like brown rice, oats, wheat and millet; dried fruit like raisins and apricots; and fish and lean chicken (without the skin).

- *Folic Acid and B12:* Folate or folic acid and Vitamin-B12 play a vital role in many bodily functions, including cell

> repair and maintenance, DNA synthesis, amino acid metabolism, and the formation of leukocytes and erythrocytes. The food sources would be vegetables like spinach, asparagus, avocados, lettuce, turnip greens, broccoli, cauliflower, beets; fruits like orange juice, pineapple juice, cantaloupe, honeydew melon, grapefruit juice, banana, raspberry, grapefruit and strawberry; legumes like moong, kidney beans, chick peas; and meat and poultry.

Most of us eat too much sodium. Limit yourself to less than 2300 mg, about one tsp of salt, every day. Reducing sodium in the diet can help lower your blood pressure.

Meeting your potassium requirement (4700 milligrams each day) by eating foods rich in potassium such as bananas and tender coconut water can also help to lower sodium intake in the body.

Portion Control

There are some simple tips for exercising portion control which I am going to share with you.

- ❑ Always eat off a small plate. You will always restrict your portions.
- ❑ Serve yourself the raw food like veggies first. It takes up more space.
- ❑ Serve rice and dal/gravy in small bowls. Try to restrict to only one helping.
- ❑ Serve all the items at one time and eat slowly till everything is over.

- If you are still hungry, take another helping of raw food or dal/gravy or yogurt. Do not reach for the staples like roti or rice.
- Ensure your salad has crunch and flavour. Use legumes and nuts in the salad for variety and taste.

My Top Five Tips for Energetic Health

- ***Eat for pleasure, control cravings and boost energy***: Your diet has a major effect on your food cravings, your stress levels, and your energy throughout the day. By making smart food choices and developing healthy eating habits, you'll find it much easier to stay slim, control cravings, and feel energetic all day long.

  Eat breakfast. Get your metabolism going in the morning by eating a healthy breakfast. Studies show that people who eat breakfast tend to weigh less than those who skip it. A solid breakfast provides energy for the day.

  Eat regularly. Going too long between meals can make you feel irritable and tired, so aim to eat something at least every three to four hours. Support your body's natural cycle of energy by eating a substantial breakfast, a nutritious lunch, a snack around 2 p.m. (to compensate for the body's natural low point that occurs around 3 each afternoon), and a light early dinner.

  Cut the junk. The ups and downs that come with eating sugary snacks and simple carbohydrates cause extreme swings in energy level and mood. Cutting out these foods can be tough, but if you can resist for several days, your cravings will subside.

- *Forget no carb, be smart carb*: Foods such as baked potatoes, whole-wheat pasta, brown rice, oatmeal, whole grain breads and bananas boost your 'feel-good' serotonin levels without a crash. They also provide plenty of fibre, so you feel full much longer. Carbs, like fats, are a vital part of a healthy diet. You should not cut them out of your diet. They give you the fuel you need to get through your day and fight fatigue. The key is to choose the right kinds of carbohydrates.

  Complex carbohydrates—the 'smart carbs'—have not been stripped of their fibre and nutrients. Because they're rich in fibre, they keep you full longer and help with weight control. Good sources of complex carbs include whole grains such as whole grain brown rice, stone ground whole wheat, millet, or quinoa, as well as beans, other legumes, fruit and vegetables.

  Simple carbohydrates—the 'bad carbs'—have been stripped of their fibre and many of their nutrients. Simple carbs lead to a dramatic spike in your blood sugar, followed by a rapid crash. These carbs are much less efficient in filling you up and keeping you energized. Simple carbs include white flour, white rice and sugary foods.

- *Don't cut out the fat*: Many women have been led to believe that dietary fat is unhealthy and contributes to weight gain. But fats are a necessary part of a healthy diet. What really matters are the types of fat you eat. So don't go no fat, go good fat.

Polyunsaturated and monounsaturated fats—the 'good fats'—contribute to your health and vitality, support your mood, help you maintain a healthy weight and improve the look of your hair, skin and nails. Monounsaturated fats are found in plant oils like canola oil, peanut oil, and olive oil, as well as avocados, nuts (like almonds, hazelnuts and pecans), and seeds (such as pumpkin, sesame). Polyunsaturated fats include Omega-3 and Omega-6 fatty acids, found in fatty fish such as salmon, herring, mackerel, anchovies and sardines. Other sources include unheated sunflower, corn, soybean, flaxseed oils and walnuts.

Saturated fat and trans fat—the 'bad fats'—increase your risk of heart disease and stroke. Saturated fats are found primarily in animal sources including red meat and whole milk dairy products. Trans fats are found in vegetable shortenings, some margarines, crackers, candies, cookies, snack foods, fried foods, baked goods, and other processed foods made with partially hydrogenated vegetable oils.

THE OIL SELECTION QUANDARY

For most women, there is always a question, which is the best and healthiest oil to use. Is sunflower oil better than olive oil? Should I use different oils in different seasons? What is this rice bran oil? So many options available in the marketplace only lead to more confusion. So let us look at some simple principles of oil selection:

- There is increasing research that blended oils with anti-oxidants have a protective anti-inflammatory effect on the heart and body as a whole.
- Anti-oxidants are proven to reduce LDL cholesterol and reduce inflammation, and hence protect the heart.
- Combinations of two oils such as safflower and rice bran is proven to be synergistic and can be blended well to give added benefits of anti-oxidation and control cholesterol, along with other measures.
- Anti-oxidation helps store oil better and also protects the integrity of the oil at high smoking points.

Oil rotation, periodically once in three months amongst the blends is also recommended by some nutritionists for the body to experience benefits of the anti-inflammatory properties of different oils.

OIL USAGE GUIDELINES

- Usage of oil must be measured, restricted to two to three teaspoons per person per day on a regular basis.
- Choose your oil wisely, based on research, anti-oxidant properties, composition and balance of MUFAs etc.
- When using any oil such as olive oil, raw in salads, always opt for the extra virgin one.

- ❑ Deep-frying once in a while for a normal healthy person is not harmful.
- ❑ Track your oil usage for the family by tagging dates on when you open a bottle or can.

Adopt healthy cooking measures like steaming and broiling to cut usage of cooking oil.

The Power of Healthy Fats

Boosts your brainpower and mood: Fats are essential to healthy brain function. They put you in a good mood and keep you mentally sharp.

Promotes healthy pregnancies: When you're pregnant, both you and your growing baby need healthy fat to feel your best. Fat is especially important to your baby's developing brain and nervous system.

Contributes to lifelong beauty: Fats are essential for vibrant and glowing skin, hair and nails. A lack of healthy fats in your diet can lead to dull, flaky skin, brittle nails, and dry or easily damaged hair.

Helps control cravings: Because fat is so dense in calories, a little goes a long way in making you feel full. Small amounts of good fats like nuts or seeds make great satisfying snacks.

Lowers the glycaemic index of foods, easing the spike in blood sugar that results from eating carbohydrates.

Helps absorb certain vitamins: Many important vitamins—

including Vitamins—A, D, E and K—are fat-soluble, meaning you need fat in your system in order to absorb them.

Focus on Foods for Strong Bones

It's important for women of all ages to eat foods that contribute to strong, healthy bones, as women have a higher risk of osteoporosis than men. Osteoporosis is largely preventable with good nutrition and exercise. After the age of 30, you stop building bone mass, but you can eat to maintain strong bones at any age. The key is to get enough of the nutrients that support bone health.

Calcium and magnesium, in combination with Vitamin-D, are vital for women's bone health. Calcium and magnesium needs are higher for people who eat the standard Western diet (high consumption of sugar, caffeine, meat and alcohol and a relatively low consumption of leafy greens and whole grains).

Calcium: The recommended daily allowance varies from 400 to 1200 mg/day. Good sources of calcium include dairy products, leafy green vegetables, oatmeal and other grains, tofu, cabbage, summer squash, green beans, garlic, and sea vegetables. Be smart about taking calcium supplements. Calcium is absorbed slowly and your body cannot take in more than 500 mg at any one time and there's no benefit in exceeding the recommended daily allowance. In fact, doing so may even harm the heart.

Magnesium: The recommended daily allowance for magnesium is 500 to 800 mg/day. Calcium only works when taken in conjunction with magnesium. Good sources of magnesium include leafy green vegetables, summer squash, broccoli, halibut, cucumber, green beans, celery, and a variety of seeds, including pumpkin, sunflower, sesame and flax seeds.

Vitamin-D: Aim for between 400 and 1000 IU (international units) daily. You can get Vitamin-D from about half an hour of direct exposure to sunlight, and from foods and supplements. Salmon is an excellent source of Vitamin-D. Other good sources include shrimp, Vitamin-D fortified milk, cod and eggs.

Add Fibre for Weight Loss

That's right—fibre benefits much more than just digestive health and all those bodily functions we'd rather not think about. Eating foods high in dietary fibre can lower your risk of heart disease, stroke and diabetes, improve the health of your skin, and even help you maintain a healthy weight.

Since fibre stays in the stomach longer than other foods, that feeling of fullness will stay with you much longer, helping you eat less. Many high-fibre foods, such as fruit and vegetables, tend to be low in calories, so adding fibre to your diet makes it easier to cut down on the calories. By regulating your blood sugar levels, fibre can help maintain your body's fat-burning capacity and regulate insulin spikes that leave you feeling drained and craving unhealthy foods.

Eating plenty of fibre can also move fat through your digestive system at a faster rate so that less of it is absorbed. When you fill up on high-fibre foods such as fruit, you'll also have more energy for exercising.

How Much Is Right?

Women aged 18 to 50: At least 25 grams of per day

Women over 50: a little less, at least 21 grams per day.

Sources of fibre: Oats, whole grains, wheat cereals, barley, flaxseed, oatmeal, beans, nuts, veggies such as carrot, celery, tomato, and fruits such as apple, berries, citrus fruits and pears.

OATS: AN OLD FRIEND, A NEW SUPER FOOD?

Oats are well-known to be a good source of soluble fibre, the type of dietary fibre linked to lower blood cholesterol and a decreased risk of diabetes. However, oats also contain a high concentration of insoluble fibre. This is true for steel-cut, old-fashioned rolled and quick-cooking oats, all of which are nutritionally similar. A diet that includes a high intake of foods providing both soluble and insoluble fibre may help prevent obesity, stroke, high blood pressure and heart disease

Benefits

The insoluble fibre in oats consists of lignin, cellulose and hemicellulose, the compounds responsible for the rigid structure of plant cell walls. In your digestive tract, the insoluble fibre you obtain from oats is not broken down and does not absorb water. Instead, it adds bulk to your stool, stimulating regular bowel movements. A diet that includes plenty of foods rich in insoluble fibre may promote digestive system health by lowering your risk of disorders like haemorrhoids, diverticular disease, constipation, intestinal ulcers, gastroesophageal reflux disease and colon cancer.

Insoluble Fibre Content

A 1/3-cup serving of uncooked oats contains 2.7 total grams of dietary fibre; of this amount, 1.3 grams are insoluble fibre and 1.4 grams are soluble fibre. Insoluble fibre is increasingly seen as the vital nutrient in promoting healthy weight loss and weight control. Oats contain about the same amount of insoluble fibre in every 1/3-cup serving as a 1/2-cup serving of cooked broccoli, 1 medium-sized raw carrot, half of a cup of applesauce, 2 medium-sized plums or half of a small, peeled mango. It is a far better source of insoluble fibre than foods like cauliflower, cucumbers, raisins, watermelon, white bread, sunflower or sesame seeds and nuts such as walnuts.

The Importance of Taste

Although we pick our foods with health in our minds, the taste of the food is critical in determining sustained changes to our diet. I recommend the use of taste and flavour enhancers like herbed salt, pepper and spices to add taste to the food preparations. I also recommend we use an approach called the healthy approach. Here's how it works.

- You want to eat a dosa for breakfast. But you need to make it healthier. So what do you do?
    - You could make the dosa batter from brown rice, but you may be using store made batter, so what do you do?
    - You could add two tablespoons of powdered oats to the dosa batter for every four dosas. This way you have immediately increased the health value while retaining the taste of the food. This is called making any dish a healthy dish.
- If you are used to eating idlis and chutney for breakfast, add on a sambar with multiple vegetables and swap coconut chutney for tomato, lentil and bell pepper chutney.
- If you eat oats with milk and sugar, swap it for cooking oats with a mix of vegetables and simple spices for a more healthy breakfast option.
- If you eat scrambled eggs and toast, swap it for a vegetable or Spanish omelette with a slice of wholewheat bread.

This can be done with any food item. If you let your imagination run riot and get creative in the kitchen, substituting unhealthy ingredients with healthy ones becomes really easy.

If you like snacks in between meals, do not reach for biscuits or chips. Try these healthy choices instead:

- Fruit dip with wholewheat and oat crackers
- A small handful of nuts rolled with dates
- An oats uttappa with vegetables

- ❑ Baby carrots and cherry tomatoes with a yoghurt dip
- ❑ A wholewheat paratha with curd
- ❑ Khakra with red pepper chutney

Eating Out healthy

Most of us manage to be good with our diets at home but slip up when we have to eat out. Here are some simple tips to eat healthy at any restaurant of your choice and enjoy any type of cuisine while still making the right food choices.

In an Italian Restaurant

- ❑ As far as possible order fresh pasta Aglio Olio, without the sauces but with plenty of vegetables and lean chicken.
- ❑ If you feel like having a sauce, opt for a red sauce on the side.
- ❑ Always take a side order of grilled vegetables or sautéed spinach.

When Ordering a Sandwich

- ❑ Add lettuce and tomato.
- ❑ Ask for wholewheat or rye bread.
- ❑ Choose mustard instead of mayonnaise.

At Chinese Restaurants

- ❑ Have brown rice instead of white rice.
- ❑ Order a side dish of steamed broccoli.
- ❑ Opt for stir fried over pan fried or deep fried.

At Fast-food Places

- ❑ Order smaller burgers.
- ❑ Have grilled chicken.
- ❑ Choose water or low-fat milk instead of ordering soft drinks.

At Pizza Places

- ❑ Ask for vegetable toppings, such as mushrooms or peppers, rather than meat toppings.
- ❑ Get wholewheat crust.
- ❑ Request half the cheese.

At Indian Restaurants

- ❑ Order fewer appetizers.
- ❑ Opt for tandoori items.
- ❑ Opt for dry vegetables and lighter tomato based gravies. rather than heavy cream based ones.
- ❑ Opt for a pulao over a biryani.

In Any Restaurant:

- ❑ Ask for salad dressing, gravy or sauce on the side and use sparingly.
- ❑ Choose main dishes that are broiled, baked, roasted or grilled, instead of deep-fried or pan-fried.
- ❑ Don't be afraid to make special requests, such as asking that something be cooked with less fat.

Enjoy Your Food

The last note I want to leave you with is to exhort you to enjoy your food. Food is not something to be feared nor an enemy to be hated. Food is very special in that it can make us happy, elevate our moods, bring a family together, mark occasions and, of course, provide us with nutrition. It is entirely up to us to make food our dear cherished friend rather than dreaded secret shame. Enjoying food consciously is the first step to eating right on a consistent basis. Healthy food can also be extremely tasty as long as we put some creativity and thought into the preparation and eating of it. With the knowledge on nutrition and the foods that can be combined for a balanced meal, set your creativity free and enjoy every meal that you make, eat or serve in your home and elsewhere.

TO SUMMARIZE

A balanced diet is key—focus on essential nutrients like calcium, iron and folates

Don't avoid any food group

Focus on fibre and protein intake is important

Eating out can be healthy too

Substitute or replace with nutrient-dense food

Every calorie is not the same

Relax and enjoy your food

WHAT'S ON YOUR PLATE?

NEW RECIPES WITH NUTRITIOUS SUBSTITUTION!

It is hard to think of new, exciting recipes all the time without compromising nutrition or taste. Most of us struggle with the eenui of the sameness in cooking. Maybe we have a repertoire of 20 breakfast dishes and an equal number of lunch and dinner menus. How can we cook creatively, exciting new dishes everyday that will also fully take care of the nutrition needs of every member of the family? Is it really that difficult?

I have put together a few recipes to show you how you can substitute any ingredient for a more nutritious option without compromising taste. I have also included more protein rich ingredients in regular food as most Indian women eat less protein than their daily requirement. These, however, are only a starting point. Once you get the hang of nutritous substitution, you will realise that you can make as many new recipes as you want by just paying a little thought to maximising nutrition from the calories we eat.

Mixed Vegetable Thalipeeth

Thalipeeth is a popular Maharashtrian breakfast made from a combination of flours such as rice and chickpeas. Here is a twist to the traditional recipe.

Ingredients

1/4 cup jowar (white millet) flour

1/4 cup bajra (black millet) flour

1/4 cup oats finely powdered

2 tbsp besan (Bengal gram flour)

2 tbsp whole wheat flour (gehun ka atta)

2 tbsp ragi (nachni/red millet) flour

1 tsp cumin seeds (jeera)

1 tsp sesame seeds (til)

1 tbsp chopped coriander (dhania)

Salt to taste

1 small onion, finely chopped

2 pinches of turmeric powder (haldi)

1/2 cup mixed boiled vegetables mashed (potatoes, beans, carrots, cauliflower, etc.)

1 tbsp ground peanut powder

Chili powder to taste

2 tbsp oil (Olive or vegetable oil)

Method

Mix all the ingredients, pour a little water and knead into a soft dough.

Divide the dough in six equal portions.

Roll out the thalipeeth between two sheets of plastic into a circle of 5' diameter—can be slightly thick.

Heat the tava, and grease it lightly with oil.

Cook the thalipeeth on both the sides using little oil till brown spots appear on it.

Serve hot with green chutney and masala curd.

Bhel Chaat

Bhel is possibly, the single most poular street food of Mumbai. Here is a way to enjoy it without compromising nutrition!

Ingredients

Half cup puffed rice or murmura

One cup moong sprouts, steamed lightly

1/2 onion, chopped

1 tomato, chopped

1/2 potato (boiled), chopped

12-15 peanuts

2 tsp lemon juice

Chaat masala as per taste

Few coriander leaves

Method

In a bowl mix puffed rice, sprouts, onions, tomato, potato and groundnut.

Squeeze lemon juice, add chaat masala and mix again.

Garnish with coriander leaves and serve immediately.

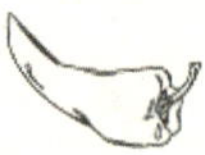

Palak Oats Moong Dal Dosa

Dosa is a universally loved dish from Tamil Nadu made from rice and lentils.Try this exciting new recipe!

Ingredients

2 bunches of palak/spinach

I cup moong dal

I cup ground oats powder

4 green chilies

I cup finely chopped onions

I bunch coriander

Few curry leaves

Salt to taste

Method

Wash and soak the moong dal for four hours.

Grind one cup of oats to a fine powder.

Finely chop the coriander and spinach. Keep aside.

Add green chillies, salt, curry leaves to the drained moong dal. Grind this to a smooth paste. Add the oats powder to the last grind and make the batter smooth.

Add the chopped onions, coriander and spinach to the batter.

Heat a dosa tava or a pan.

Pour one big tablespoon of the batter on the pan.

Quickly spread the batter outwards to the edge of the pan.

Add a little oil to the edge of the dosa and few drops on the top to enable it to fry.

Keep this on high flame for about two minutes till the corners of the dosa leave the surface of the pan.

Now remove the dosa from the pan and place it on a serving plate.

Serve with a vegetable sambar or chutney of your choice.

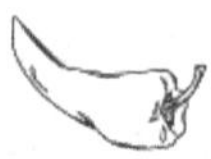

Paratha Pizza

All across the north of India, the paratha is the king! But kids of today want pizza which is a western import made of refined flour. Here's a way to keep moms and kids happy!

Ingredients for the Paratha

3-4 tbsp oil for frying parathas

1 and 1/2 cup wheat flour (atta)

1/2 tsp carom seeds (ajwain)

1/2 tsp cumin seeds (jeera)

1 tsp dried mango powder (amchur)

2 tbsp oil

1/2 tsp salt

Cold water to knead the dough

Method

In a large bowl mix wheat flour, carom seeds, cumin seeds, dried mango powder, salt and oil. Add cold water little by little and knead the whole mixture into a smooth, soft dough (like chapati dough).

Cover and set it aside for 15-20 minutes. After that, divide it into eight equal-sized flattened balls and keep those aside.

Take two flattened balls and roll out into rotis.

Place one roti on the top of the other and seal the edges. Roll out again with a soft hand.

Heat tawa or griddle, roast each paratha the usual way till both sides are done. Add little oil on both sides of the paratha.

Ingredients for the Pizza Topping

1 tsp oil

1 tsp finely chopped onion

1 tsp finely chopped garlic

2 tbsp finely chopped capsicum

2 tsp finely chopped tomato

2 tsp corn kernels

2 tsp chopped mushrooms

1/2 tsp finely chopped green chillies

Salt to taste

1/2 tsp black pepper

2-3 tbsp tomato puree

Grated cheese (preferably Mozzarella)

Method

Heat oil in a pan. Put chopped onion, garlic, capsicum, tomato, corn kernels, mushrooms and finely chopped green chillies in it.

Sauté the ingredients well.

After a few minutes, add salt, black pepper and tomato puree. Mix well.

Add oil in another pan and heat a pre-cooked parantha on both sides. Put the vegetable mixture and grated cheese on it.

Let it cook on slow flame for 3-4 mins till it turns crispy and the grated cheese melts.

You can also put the parathas with topping in an oven preheated to 180 degrees Celsius.

Tofu Red Pepper Scramble on Whole Wheat Bread

For those of us pure vegetarians, a yummy shot of protein with anti-oxidants aplenty!

Ingredients

400g firm tofu

1/2 cup white onion, diced

1/2 cup button mushrooms, chopped

1/2 cup red pepper, diced

1 tsp minced garlic

1 tsp red chili powder

1/4 tsp turmeric (optional)

1 tbsp olive oil

1 tsp whole wheat flour mixed in 1/4 cup milk or water

Method

Grate the tofu through a large-sieved grater.

Heat the oil in a pan. Add the garlic, turmeric powder and chili powder.

Add the peppers and mushrooms on a high flame and cook till the mushrooms lose no more water.

Add the tofu and cook for 3-4 minutes. Add salt to taste.

Add the flour-milk/water mixture and cook for a couple of minutes till it all comes together and thickens a bit.

Garnish with cilantro leaves.

Cilantro Chutney

One bunch cilantro leaves cleaned and cut

2-3 green chilies

1 onion chopped

Juice of one lemon

Blend the first three ingredients in a blender-grinder. Add the lemon juice and salt to taste.

To Assemble the Sandwich

2 slices whole wheat bread

2 tsp cilantro chutney

Method

Take the bread and toast it to a medium heat.

Apply the cilantro chutney on one side of both slices.

Place both slices down and put the scrambled tofu on the cilantro side and make an open-faced sandwich.

Serve immediately.

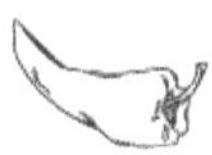

Steamed Dahi Vadas

A much loved snack with all its flavour minus the oil!

I cup ural dal soaked for two hours along with I tsp moong dal

4 dried red chillies

Salt to taste

For the Dahi

I cup yoghurt

I/4 of a coconut grated

3 green chilies

Method

First grind the coconut and green chilies and add to the yoghurt along with a bit of salt.

Then grind all the ingredients for the vada with just a little water to make a coarse paste. This is your batter.

Take a saucepan and boil one litre of water.

Drop spoonfuls of batter into the water and cook till they float like dumplings.

Remove with a slotted spoon, squeeze and add to pre-prepared dahi.

Season with mustard seeds, curry leaves and a pinch of asafoetida.

Garnish with cilantro and serve cold.

Peas and Almond Pulao with Brown Rice

A rich and nutritious rice preparation!

Ingredients

1 cup brown basmati rice

2 tbsp vegetable oil

6-8 cups water

1 small onion

1 tsp salt

1 tsp cumin seed

1/4 cup frozen or fresh peas

1 tsp black pepper

1 stick cinnamon

2 bay leaves

1/2 cup toasted almonds

Method

Wash and drain the rice three times to remove the starch.

Bring water to boil after adding 1 tsp ghee, 2 star anise and salt to the water.

Add the rice and let it come to a boil.

Cook further for 15 minutes. Turn off the flame and cover and let it cook for about 15 minutes till the rice is fully done.

Drain the water, remove the star anise and cool the rice.

With burner on high, heat oil in a heavy pan. Add onion and cook until translucent (not brown), for about 2 minutes.

Add cumin seed, black pepper, cinnamon and bay leaf and stir for one minute.

Add the peas along with salt and cook for about 5 to 7 minutes.

Turn the flame to low and add the cooked rice.

Turn off the flame and gently mix. Add toasted almonds on top. Serve.

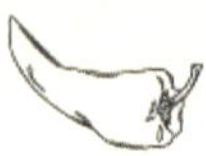

Corn Cilantro Chickpea Fritters (Makai Vadi)

Super healthy and super yummy!

Ingredients

1/2 cup cooked and crushed corn

1 small bunch finely chopped cilantro

1 cup besan (gram flour)

2 cups water

Salt to taste

1 tsp chili powder

Method

Heat the water to boiling and turn down the flame.

Add the chickpea flour with salt and chilli powder and stir till no lumps form.

As the batter begins to thicken, add the corn and cilantro and cook for about 2 minutes.

Take a one-inch deep pan and grease it on the sides. Add the cooked batter. Cool.

Cover with cling wrap and refrigerate for 2 hours.

Remove. Cut into squares and sauté or shallow fry in a pan till golden brown.

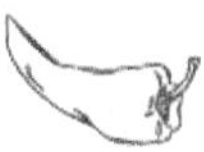

Amaranth Leaves in Yoghurt Curry (Lal Math Moru Koottan)

So tasty, even the vegetable averse love it!

Ingredients

1 bunch amaranth leaves, cut and finely chopped

1 cup yoghurt, thinned into 2 cups with water

1/2 cup grated coconut

1 tsp cumin seeds

2 green chillies

Method

Grind the coconut, cumin seeds and green chilies with a little yoghurt.

Mix in the rest of the thinned yoghurt.

Cook the amaranth separately and lightly mash with a spoon.

Drain water and add salt to taste.

Take a deep pan and add 1 tsp oil and heat.

Add mustard seeds, curry leaves and one red chili till it sputters.

Add the yoghurt mixture on a low flame and stir till no lumps are formed.

Add the leaves and cook for about 5 minutes. The colour will be red.

Turn the gas off and serve with rice or rotis.

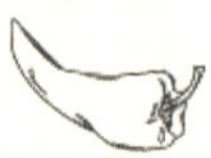

Weight and Watch!

I have been there, done that and failed—tried every new diet in town, obsessed over the numbers, weighed myself every morning before water, after ablution, jumped on every new bandwagon that promised weight loss, better shape, quicker results—and never felt well. Even the rare times I lost weight, I piled it back on.

Then I started delving into researches on nutrition and started speaking to experts: dieticians, trainers, naturopaths, bariatric surgeons, Ayurveda doctors, and realized that there is just too much information there, a lot of it conflicting, some of it confusing and most of it is just too complicated.

When I sat down to sift through the material, and put down a framework that most of us can work with, I realized that it is really not just about adopting a new diet or a better exercise regimen—it is about making those changes to one's lifestyle that make good health sustainable.

There are so many ways in which weight is measured: weighing scales, body mass index, fat percentage, but what is most important is to have a sense of well-being—to be full of energy and have the ability to live life to the fullest without niggling aches and pains. These are things we seldom think about in our single-minded quest to lose those kilos and inches, and hence I decided to personally adopt the SLIMZ approach to attaining an optimum weight for wellness.

SLIMZ stands for the following:

S: Simplify
L: Less Fads
I: Inch by Inch

M: Menu Plan
Z: Zen and Zone

S: Simplify

We need to stop complicating it so much. No one, in a regular life on a regular day can sit and calculate to a precise degree how much carbohydrates, proteins, fats she consumes on a long-term or sustainable basis. The important thing is, if you want to lose weight, *eat less*. But focus on your meal being a balanced meal, focus on protein, fibre, vegetables and fruits.

Ensure you eat a high-fibre, high protein breakfast every day. Eating a healthy breakfast helps to maintain sugar and metabolism levels, diminishing hunger pangs. This ensures that one is not tempted to snack on sugary treats.

L: Less Fads

Any diet that promises weight loss will eventually ask you to cut those calories down. Fad diets sound exotic because they often promote a totally different way of eating from what you are used to. However, therein lies the problem, because it is the very reason why these fad diets are not sustainable. Very often, they may provide short-term weight loss, but promote cravings and cause the weight of the person to fluctuate, which is actually much worse metabolically.

The only way to approach weight loss is to look at how to stay nutritionally well-balanced while creating a calorie deficit. So make a vow to pursue no more fly by night diet plans, but to stick to small changes that can be effected over a period of time and that can result in substantial benefits.

I: Inch By Inch

This is the most important aspect of this approach. Changes to diet and exercise have to be gradual and sustainable. The weight loss must be accompanied by inch loss as well but just like Rome was not built in a day, it must be kept in mind that changes in exercise too must be built up gradually.

Begin with moderate exercise. Instead of trying to change your entire life with an intense weight loss plan, start small. Make a commitment to get yourself moving for at least 10-15 minutes each day for 30 days straight.

If you're already a runner or a cyclist or a swimmer, then begin a very modest programme of resuming that exercise. Otherwise, walking in the park or on a treadmill, hiking, cycling on a cycling machine, rowing, or something similar exercise would work. Mixing it up is a great idea, alternating different exercises on different days. The actual exercise you do doesn't matter, as long as you get moving.

I repeat: Start out really easy. People tend to start with a lot of enthusiasm, and then burn out, skip a workout or two, and then the plan has already failed. Start slow but do it every day. Go for about half of what you think you can do. You can always add on more later.

Set aside some time to do this every day. If you've had success working out in the morning before, use that time. Otherwise, do it right after work.

Strength training for inch loss: Don't do anything too tough in the first couple of weeks. Just some push-ups, crunches, lunges, squats, with no weights. That might sound like too little but the key, again, is to start out slow.

If you are feeling resistance to exercising, just tell yourself that you have to lace up your shoes and get out of the door. How long you do it doesn't matter, even 15 minutes is good. Recent research has showed that even moderate exercise is the most potent weapon in the fight against bad lifestyle-induced diseases.

M: Menu Plan

To start eating for weight loss, three things are most important. The first is to plan your meals through the day, the second is replacement. Replace low-nutrition foods with high-nutrition ones and the third is portion control.

Replace high sugar, fatty and greasy foods with healthier options. Take a look at what you eat, and try to slowly replace the greasier and fattier foods with healthier alternatives. If you cook fried chicken, try baked instead. If you eat burgers, try a patty in a wholewheat wrap. If you eat puris, replace with theplas.

First, focus on making your breakfast your healthiest meal. Include easy but super healthy options like oatmeal, ready-to-eat cereals with a fruit and some sprouts or an egg.

Eat smaller meals, more frequently. Once you start getting used to less fatty foods, try eating smaller portions, and eating five to six times a day instead of just three big meals. This requires a meal plan, so you can include variety with nutrition-dense foods. A good schedule is to eat breakfast, then a mid-morning snack, then a small early lunch, then an afternoon snack, then a small, light dinner.

Make sure that your snacks are healthy ones. Good ones include fruits, nuts, khakras, salad bhel, yoghurt, cut-up veggies with hummus or baba ghanoush. It's important that you gradually reduce your portions, and learn to eat only until you're satiated, not until you're bursting. This is the most effective change for sustainable good health and weight loss

Z: Zen and Zone

Be relaxed about your approach but determined about your goals. Get into a Zen frame of mind about your diet and exercise rather than constantly ruing the fact that you have to think about what you eat. If you accept the need to get healthy and fit happily, the weight loss follows.

Zone out once in a while. Don't be too tough on yourself. Have a cheat day every week, to indulge in one favourite dish in moderation. But keep it to one dish and do it with a plan. While spontaneous eating may be fun, it usually throws the whole meal plan out of gear.

The important and most vital thing to remember is that usually there is no end to a fitness or weight loss journey. Once an ideal weight is attained, the same approach is required to maintain that weight. Hence, make the changes according to the SLIMZ approach to ensure that the changes are lasting and sustainable.

SLIMZ APPROACH

S: Simplify
L: Less Fads
I: Inch by Inch
M: Menu Plan
Z: Zen and Zone

7

A Hormonious Life

You are at work, reviewing a monthly performance, and you find that one of your team members has messed up an important task. You suddenly have a meltdown moment and tear him apart. After you calm down, you know that everyone in your team is shaking his or her head and saying 'menopausal crazies' and you start wondering, 'Oh God, is this menopause?'

So, what is menopause?

Menopause is when we turn moody, screechy, when everything annoys us, our bones creak and we feel as bloated as the back of a truck. Ok, ok, I'm kidding!

Menopause is a normal, natural event—defined as the final menstrual period and usually confirmed when a woman has missed her periods for twelve consecutive months (in the absence of other obvious causes). The term 'menopause' comes from the Greek words 'meno' (month) and 'pause' (to end). Thus, it literally means permanent physiological or natural cessation of the menstrual cycle. Menopause is associated with reduced functioning of the ovaries due to ageing, resulting in lower levels of oestrogen and other hormones. It marks the permanent end of fertility. Menopause occurs, on an average, between ages 45-55. The term 'pre-menopause' refers to the phase of life that precedes menopause. For many women, it is a time to reassess their health.

So what are the changes that you should expect around this time?

Each woman's menopause experience is different. Many who undergo natural menopause report no physical changes at all during the peri-menopause years except irregular menstrual periods that eventually stop when they reach menopause. Other changes may include hot flushes, difficulty in sleeping, lack of memory, mood disturbances, vaginal dryness and weight gain. Not all these changes are hormone-related, and some, such as hot flushes and memory problems, tend to get resolved after menopause. Maintaining a healthy lifestyle during this time of transition is essential for your health and can cushion you against some of these changes.

Hot Flushes

Hot flushes refer to the state of feeling flushed followed by feeling cold. It is the most common menopause-related discomfort. Although their exact cause still isn't fully understood, hot flushes are thought to be the result of changes in the hypothalamus, the part of the brain that regulates the body's temperature. If the hypothalamus mistakenly senses that a woman is too warm, it starts a chain of events to cool her down. Blood vessels near the surface of the skin begin to dilate (enlarge), increasing blood flow to the surface in an attempt to deflect body heat. This produces a red, flushed look on the face and neck in light-skinned women. It may also make a woman perspire to cool the body down. The heart may beat faster, and women may sense that rapid heartbeat. A cold chill often follows a hot flash. A few women experience only the chill.

But the good news is that hot flushes are temporary and usually last a few months only, though in some cases they may last up to two years. They are often accompanied by loss of libido, vaginal dryness, mood swings and irregular periods, either shorter, lighter periods or heavier periods with flooding.

Although the available treatments for hot flushes do not cure them, they do offer relief. Even without treatment hot flushes usually fade away eventually, and no treatment is necessary unless they become really bothersome. A few women have only an occasional hot flush. There are a number of low-risk coping strategies and lifestyle changes that may be helpful for managing hot flushes, but if they get very disruptive, prescription therapy may be considered. These include hormone replacement therapy with oestrogen progesterone or oestrogen cyproterone acetate combinations.

Dry Eyes

After menopause, some women report chronically dry and scratchy eyes, often along with light sensitivity, blurred vision, or swollen or reddened eyelids—a condition called chronic dry eye. Tearing can also be a symptom, because the eye produces more watery tears to compensate, although these tears don't lubricate the eyes the way healthy tears do. Sometimes, the condition is caused by certain diseases (such as Sjögren's Syndrome) or drugs (such as allergy medications and anti-depressants). In mild cases, over-the-counter artificial tear drops or gels can help. Drinking more water and taking Omega-3 supplements may also be beneficial. More severe cases may require prescription medication or plugging tear ducts to keep tears in the eyes longer. It is wise to visit an eye doctor when you hit menopause and from then on, at least once a year.

Receding Gums

Your dental health and the health of your bones are closely related. So although problems with the teeth and gum may be more common at and after menopause, don't think of them as 'normal.' With bone loss, the tooth sockets in your jaw deteriorate, leading to receding gums and exposed roots that make you sensitive to cold. Take good care of your teeth and your bones. Get regular dental check-ups, and follow your dentist's advice about flossing, brushing and rinsing. Check your Vitamin-D level. A lot of Indian women have Vitamin-D deficiency this could lead to osteoporosis if neglected.

Aches and Pains

Menopause and loss of oestrogen make your bones more fragile. There is a loss of bone strength that makes you vulnerable to broken bones. Although women start losing bone in their 30s, the process speeds up after menopause. Osteoporosis is a 'silent' disease, that is, you may not know you have it until you have a broken bone. Testing for osteoporosis with a bone mineral density test is usually recommended for women at the age of 65. If you are less than 65 and have what's called a 'fragility fracture', that is, a bone break typical of weakened bones (often in the wrist), that indicates you have osteoporosis. Usually fractures occur because of an external injury but when your bones are weak, they may break with even regular daily activities because they are fragile. This is called fragility fracture.

As a general practice, good nutrition and exercise goes a long way in maintaining healthy bones.

Heart Ailments

It is a little-known fact that more women get heart disease than cancer and heart health is extremely important for women. We shall discuss this in detail in chapter The Heart Truth.

Weight Gain

Although published literature says that there is no connection between menopause and weight gain, many women do gain weight and fat gets redistributed after menopause. Altered hormones may lead to slowing down of the metabolic rate; the body's need for calories reduces, but often lifestyles that include frequent eating out do not change. Also a lot of women resort to comfort eating around this age. It is good to be watchful and keep the weight under control as obesity itself may drive lifestyle diseases like diabetes, high blood pressure, compromised heart health, weak knees and bones. Hence, it is good to eat healthy, exercise regularly and sleep well to maintain your weight and prevent a host of lifestyle diseases.

Vaginal Dryness/GSM

Vaginal dryness is extremely common during menopause. It's just one of a collection of symptoms known as the Genitourinary Syndrome of Menopause (GSM) that involves changes to the vulvovaginal area as well as to the urethra and bladder. These changes can lead to vaginal dryness, pain during intercourse, urinary urgency and, sometimes, more frequent bladder infections.

These body changes and symptoms are usually the result of decreased oestrogen. However, decreased oestrogen is not the only cause of vaginal dryness. It is important to stop using soap and powder on the vulva, fabric softeners on your underwear, and disposable panty liners and pads. Vaginal moisturizers and lubricants may help. Persistent vaginal dryness and painful intercourse should be evaluated by a doctor. If it is determined to be a symptom of menopause, vaginal dryness can be treated with low-dose vaginal oestrogen. Regular sexual activity can help preserve vaginal function by increasing blood flow to the genital region and helping maintain the size of the vagina. Without sexual activity and oestrogen, the vagina can become smaller and dryer.

Headache

Suddenly, you may find you are losing interest in sex. Intercourse is becoming more and more painful and you find yourself feigning a headache every other night. You may be experiencing a lowered libido because of menopause and you need to be able to correct it. You may be having genuine menopausal headaches and insomnia which may be driving fatigue contributing to loss of interest in sex.

However, there are many reasons for sleep disturbances besides menopausal night sweats (simply, hot flushes at night). Your sleep disturbances may be caused by factors that affect many women in their late 40s and 50s such as sleep-disordered breathing (known as sleep apnoea), restless legs syndrome, stress, anxiety, depression, painful chronic illnesses, and even some medications. Sleep apnoea is a condition where, for many reasons ranging from a plump neck to respiratory difficulties, there are periods of sleep when your brain temporarily does not get sufficient oxygen. It could manifest as sudden snoring, a feeling of constant tiredness and even occasionally falling asleep during the day time unbeknownst to oneself.

Restless legs is a condition where, due to unknown reasons, poor circulation or a feeling of fatigue, you tend to thrash your legs constantly when you sleep. This too leads to sense of fatigue and poor rest.

Any treatment should first focus on improving your sleep routine—regular hours of sleeping each night, and avoiding getting too warm while sleeping, Excessive heat and warmth can trigger hot flushes and night sweats and interrupt quality of sleep. Avoid stimulants such as caffeine and dark chocolate that may keep you awake. When lifestyle changes fail to alleviate sleep disturbances, your clinician could refer you to a sleep centre to rule out sleep-related disorders before initiating prescription medicine. If your sleep disturbance is related solely to hot flushes, hormone therapy is likely to help.

Women at increased risk of hormonal headaches during peri-menopause are those who have already had a history of headaches influenced by hormones, such as those who suffered headaches around their periods (so-called menstrual migraines) or while taking oral contraceptives. Hormonal headaches typically stop when menopause is reached and hormone levels are consistently low. Most headaches do not require treatment or can be treated with non-prescription pain medications. Some headaches, however, can be serious. More serious headaches, including migraines, may require prescription drugs.

There are no clear-cut evidences linking low libido to menopause. There are also women who report a higher sex drive post menopause. Sometimes, the fatigue and tiredness from other symptoms of menopause may reduce your sexual desire. Find ways to keep your relationship with your partner happy and conversations around sex open. There is no acceptable frequency or correctness. Sex is a part of a loving, fulfilling relationship and should be nurtured as such.

Hair Loss and Thinning

Menopause often triggers thinning of the hair and female pattern hair loss in women. It is important to consult a dermatologist immediately to seek advice for controlling the same.

Lack of Memory and Ability to Concentrate

Difficulty in concentrating and remembering are common complaints during peri-menopause and the years right after menopause. Some data imply that even though there is a trend towards memory loss during the menopause transition, memory after the transition is as good as it was before. Memory problems may be more related to normal ageing, mood swings and other factors than to any organic cause in the body. Maintaining an extensive social network, remaining physically and mentally active, consuming a healthy diet, not smoking and consuming alcohol in moderation may all help prevent memory loss. Aim for normal cholesterol levels, normal weight and normal blood pressure to help protect your brain.

Depression and Mood Swings

Many women report symptoms of moodiness, depression, anxiety, stress and a decreased sense of well-being during perimenopause. Women with a history of clinical depression or a history of Pre-menstrual Syndrome (PMS) or post-partum depression seem to be particularly vulnerable to recurrent depression during perimenopause, as are women who report significant stress, sexual dysfunction, physical inactivity or hot flushes. It is also the time of life when women are handling more roles and responsibilities and dealing with difficult situations like parenting teenagers, grappling with demanding jobs of husbands who are at the peak of their careers and so on. The empty nest syndrome may also trigger depression and anxiety.

It has been suggested that mood disorders are related to erratic fluctuations in oestrogen levels, but limited data exists on why this occurs. Anti-depressants are the primary pharmacologic treatment for menopause-associated depression. Menopause hormone therapy and hormonal contraceptives, while intended to help with irregular periods and symptoms thereof, are sometimes prescribed to alleviate mood disorders too. This is known as an off-label therapy and may especially help women with concurrent hot flushes.

I will discuss depression in detail in a subsequent chapter in this book.

Does Hormone Replacement Therapy Work?

There is much controversy surrounding hormone replacement therapy and yet, it has a place in the treatment of severe menopausal symptoms.

Hormone replacement therapies are the prescription drugs used most often to treat hot flushes and Genitourinary Syndrome of Menopause (GSM), which includes vaginal dryness. For hot flushes, hormones are given in pills, patches, sprays, gels, or a vaginal ring that deliver hormones throughout the body—known as 'systemic' therapy. For genitourinary symptoms, hormones are given in creams, pills or rings that are inserted into the vagina.

Systemic hormones include oestrogen—either the same or similar to the oestrogen the body produces naturally—and progestogen which includes progesterone and the progestogen the body produces naturally or a similar compound. Systemic hormones are very effective for hot flushes and have other benefits such as protecting your bones. They also carry risks, such as blood clots and breast cancer. The breast cancer risk usually doesn't arise until after about five years with oestrogen-progesterone therapy or after seven years with oestrogen alone. For this reason, HRT is not widely prescribed these days and women are given psychological counselling and treated with topicals. Topicals are the term given to medicines which are used as applications like creams, gels, lotions etc and can alleviate symptoms effectively.

Vaginal oestrogen therapy is a topical therapy for GSM after menopause is administered in the vagina and is effective for both moisturizing and rebuilding tissue. Very little goes into the blood so the risks of cancer are far lower.

Friends and Support Groups

Menopause is a difficult time for a lot of women. Having your friends around you, a supportive family and a healthy social network, all go a long way in making this transition easy for women. Try to nurture these relationships so you can step into the next phase of your life with the best health and confidence that you can possibly have.

TO SUMMARIZE

Menopause can be highly symptomatic

Hot flushes, mood swings, headaches are commonplace

Consult your doctor for bone check-up, dry eyes and vaginal dryness

Keep a tab on your diet and lifestyle

Menopause Symptoms

- ❑ Heart pounding or racing
- ❑ Hot flushes

- ❑ Night sweats
- ❑ Insomnia
- ❑ Memory lapses
- ❑ Depression
- ❑ Vaginal dryness
- ❑ Dry eyes
- ❑ Bone pain
- ❑ Hair loss and thinning
- ❑ Palpitations

8

Be My Baby

Anita is an extremely successful mid-level manager in a multinational firm. She has been working since she graduated from business school, for close to eight years. She got married three years ago, when she turned 30, and she and her husband Arun have been trying to conceive for the last two years, with no success. The word IVF really scares them as they know two couples who have been traumatized by the process.

Anita and her husband are not alone on this journey. Fertility and the process of making a baby have somehow got narrowed down in popular jargon to just IVF. But fertility and infertility are complex subjects that need to be understood a little more in detail.

Let's start with the basic question: How does one get pregnant?

This seems like such a silly question, right? One gets pregnant when a woman has an unprotected intercourse with a man ... Duh! But it is important to remember that the process of getting pregnant involves a series of steps and a problem with any of these steps could lead to difficulties in conception. Simplistically put the four steps are:

- A woman's body must release an egg from one of her ovaries (ovulation).
- A man's sperm must join with the egg along the way (fertilize).
- The fertilized egg must go through a fallopian tube toward the uterus (womb).
- The fertilized egg must attach to the inside of the uterus (implantation).

Infertility may result from a problem with any or several of these steps.

So when should one approach a doctor for infertility?

Most couples should consult a doctor after a year of unprotected intercourse and attempts to conceive unsuccessfully. This is the main sign of infertility. If the woman is over thirty-five and hasn't conceived after trying for six months or has an irregular menstrual cycle, it's best to see a doctor as soon as possible. Remember that the man should be evaluated, too. Male infertility is just as common as female infertility.

Infertility Incidence

In all cases of infertility, the rough split is believed to be a problem with the man 40 per cent of the time, a problem with the woman 40 per cent of the time, a problem with both ten per cent of the time, while the cause for the remaining ten per cent is unknown. Male infertility can be more easily tested and should be done from the beginning as the woman is being evaluated.

The male produces the sperm, which then travels up to the female's uterus to combine with the egg to form a union and subsequently an embryo. Problems in male fertility could be due to any one of the four processes below:

Low sperm count: The number of sperms produced in the male might be very low. Then the chances of sperm and egg union become lower.

Poor sperm motility: In some cases, the sperms are poorly motile and cannot move and swim effectively. This can affect chances of conception.

Malformed sperm: This is usually congenital or due to acquired illnesses like varicocoele (increased size of veins on the testicles).

Blocked sperm ducts: This could again be congenital or a partial block due to inflammation of the sperm ducts due to infections. Sometimes blocked ducts can be reversed by surgery.

Flaw in the movement of the sperm: This may be caused by the shape of the sperm. Sometimes injuries or other damage to the genital system block the sperm.

Testicular problems: Inflammation after mumps or similar conditions or injury, enlarged testicular blood vessels, viral infection like mumps which causes orchitis or inflammation of the testes can all impact fertility.

Sometimes a man is born with the problems that affect his sperm. Often they crop up later in life due to illness or injury. For example, tuberculosis, gonorrhoea, cystic fibrosis etc. often cause infertility in men.

So what increases a man's risk of infertility?

A man's sperm is affected by his overall health and lifestyle. Some factors that may reduce the health or number of sperm include heavy alcohol use, certain drugs like anti-depressants, environmental toxins like lead, smoking cigarettes, serious conditions like kidney disease, radiation treatment and chemotherapy for cancer, chronic exposure to heat or, anecdotally, even consistent use of tight underwear.

Female Infertility

40 per cent of infertility issues involve infertility in the female. A normally fertile woman produces eggs in the ovaries. These eggs are generally transported by the fallopian tubes to the uterus where the union with the sperm happens. The most common causes of female infertility are three-fold:

- Irregular ovulation (release of eggs)
- Blocked fallopian tubes
- Abnormalities in uterus

Most cases of female infertility are caused by problems with ovulation. Without ovulation, there are no eggs to be fertilized. Some signs that a woman is not ovulating normally include irregular or absent menstrual periods. Ovulation difficulties are often caused by polycystic ovarian syndrome (PCOS). PCOS is a hormone imbalance problem which can interfere with normal ovulation. PCOS is the most common cause of female infertility. Primary ovarian insufficiency (POI) is another cause of ovulation problems. POI occurs when a woman's ovaries stop working normally before she is 40. It is not the same as early menopause.

Blocked fallopian tubes occur due to pelvic inflammatory disease, endometriosis or surgery for an ectopic pregnancy, which is a pregnancy where the embryo is stuck in the tube. Sometimes, a woman may be born with only one tube, which could reduce her chances of fertility.

Abnormalities of the uterus could by physical and congenital, due to presence of lumps in the uterus and cervix called fibroids and, sometimes, just an unexplained hostile environment.

Many of these issues are caused by external or internal factors, which could include advancing age, stress, poor diet, excessive athletic training, being overweight or underweight, smoking, excessive alcohol use, sexually transmitted infections (STIs) like chlamydia, gonorrhoea or syphilis and, as discussed earlier, health problems that cause hormonal changes such as polycystic ovarian syndrome and primary ovarian insufficiency.

It is important to remember that a woman's best child-bearing years are from her early 20s to very early 30s. After 35, the chances of conception reduce. This, in the context of the modern woman, is very important as demands of career often delays the decision to start a family. You can extract and freeze your egg if you so wish, to balance career and family, but the ability to have a baby depends on other health factors too, like your overall health and specifically genital health at the time of implantation and hence, just freezing may not be enough.

About one-third of couples in which the woman is over 35 have fertility problems. Ageing decreases a woman's chances of having a baby in the following ways:

- The ovaries become less able to release eggs.
- The woman has a smaller number of eggs left.
- The eggs are not as healthy.
- Likelihood of health conditions that can cause fertility problems increases.
- The woman is more likely to have a miscarriage.

It must be remembered that these trends are based on statistics and may not be true in every woman's case. But all the factors must be kept in mind while planning a baby.

First Steps to Conception

If you are trying to conceive, the first step is to be aware of your menstrual cycle and the changes that happen to your body during that time. It helps to know when you are fertile.

There are four ways to track your fertile times:

1. Calendar method (most commonly used)
2. Basal body temperature method
3. Cervical mucus method (ovulation method)
4. Ultrasound method (at a doctor's clinic)

The Calendar Method

The Calendar method is based on the menstrual cycle.

The average menstrual cycle lasts 28 days. But normal cycles can vary from 21-35 days. Ovulation is a step of the female menstrual cycle whereby a mature ovarian follicle (part of the ovary) discharges a ripe egg. The amount of time before ovulation occurs is different in every woman and can even be different from month to month in the same woman, varying from 13-20 days. Learning about this part of the cycle is important because it is the starting point of the reproduction cycle for women. In women, where there is no fertilisation of the egg or ovum with the sperm, they will usually have a period within 14 to 16 days. To find out your ovulation time, record your menstrual cycle on a calendar for 8-12 months. The first day of your period is Day 1. Circle Day 1 on the calendar. The length of your cycle may vary from month to month. So write down the total number of days it lasts each time. Using this record, you can find the days you are most fertile in the months ahead:

To find out the first day when you are most fertile, subtract 18 from the total number of days in your shortest cycle. Take this new number and count ahead that many days from the first day of your next period. Draw an X through this date on your calendar. The X marks the first day you're likely to be fertile.

For example, if your cycle is 28 days, you will subtract 18 from 28 which is 10. If the first day of your period is the first, count 10 days ahead, so 11th will be your first fertile day.

To find out the last day when you are most fertile, subtract 11 from the total number of days in your longest cycle. Take this new number and count ahead that many days from the first day of your next period. Draw an X through this date on your calendar. The time between the two Xs is your most fertile window.

So if your longest cycle is 31 days, you will subtract 11 from 31 and arrive at 20, so the last fertile day is the 21st. So your most fertile window is 11th to 21st of that month.

This method should always be used along with other fertility awareness methods such as measuring your temperature or mild discharge experienced by some women during ovulation, especially if your cycles are not always of the same length.

The Menstrual Cycle

Day 1 starts with the first day of your period. This occurs after hormone levels drop at the end of the previous cycle, signalling blood and tissues lining the uterus (womb) to break down and shed from the body. Bleeding lasts about five days.

Day 7 the bleeding has stopped. Leading up to this time, hormones cause fluid-filled pockets called follicles to develop in the ovaries. Each follicle contains a potential egg.

Between Day 7 and 11, one follicle will continue to develop and reach maturity. The lining of the uterus starts to thicken, waiting for a fertilized egg to implant there. The lining is rich in blood and nutrients.

Around Day 14 (in a twenty-eight-day cycle), hormones cause the mature follicle to burst and release an egg from the ovary a process called ovulation.

Over the next few days, the egg travels down the fallopian tube towards the uterus. If a sperm unites with the egg here, the fertilized egg will continue down the fallopian tube and attach to the lining of the uterus.

If the egg is not fertilized, hormone levels will drop around Day 25. This signals the beginning of the next menstrual cycle. The egg will break apart and be shed with the next period.

The Basal Body Temperature Method

The basal body temperature is your temperature at rest as soon as you wake up in the morning. A woman's basal body temperature rises slightly with ovulation. So by recording this temperature daily for several months, you'll be able to predict your most fertile days.

Basal body temperature differs slightly from woman to woman. Anywhere from 96-98 degree Fahrenheit (35.55-36.66 degree Celcius) orally is average before ovulation. After ovulation, most women have an oral temperature of 97-99 degree Fahrenheit (36.1-37.2 degree Celsius). The rise in temperature can be a sudden jump or a gradual climb over a few days.

Usually a woman's basal body temperature rises by only 0.4-0.8 degree Fahrenheit. To detect this tiny change, women must use a basal body thermometer. These thermometers are very sensitive, but very difficult to procure. The rise in temperature doesn't show exactly when the egg is released. But almost all women ovulate within three days after their temperatures spike. Body temperature stays at the higher level until your period starts.

You are most fertile and most likely to get pregnant from 2-3 days before your temperature hits the highest point (ovulation), and 12-24 hours after ovulation.

A man's sperm can live for up to three days in a woman's body. The sperm can fertilize an egg at any point during that time. So if you have unprotected sex a few days before ovulation, there is a chance of becoming pregnant.

Many factors can affect basal body temperature. To get the most useful chart you should take your temperature every morning at about the same time. Several causes that can alter your temperature include:

- Drinking alcohol the night before
- Smoking cigarettes the night before
- Getting a poor night's sleep
- Having a fever
- Doing any activity in the morning before you take your temperature including going to the bathroom, having a cup of tea or even talking on the phone

The Cervical Mucus Method

This is a difficult method for women to track as it depends on the perception of dryness or lubrication as experienced by a woman. It is not reliable or recommended.

The Ultrasound Method

This is an extremely accurate method as a doctor can actually track the release of the egg.

Tackling Fertility Issues

If you are having fertility issues, your gynaecologist will treat you or at some stage can refer you to a fertility specialist. The specialist will need to test both you and your partner to find out where the problem lies. Depending on the issue, your doctor might recommend treatment. About nine in ten cases of infertility can be treated with drugs or surgery. Don't delay seeing your doctor as age also affects the success rates of these treatments. For some couples, adoption offers a way to share their love for a child and build a family.

Ways to Boost Egg Quality

There are some lifestyle changes, which when adopted for a period of six to nine months, can boost egg quality. Some of them are:

- *Revamping your diet:* Try to get rid of foods that cause inflammation, including refined sugar, some preservatives and nitrates, excess of simple omega-6 fatty acids and trans fats. Studies show that chronic inflammation decreases the cells' ability to respond to hormonal cues. Inflammation plays a role in diabetes and Polycystic Ovarian Syndrome (PCOS).
- *Working with a dietician*: Hormonal health may be improved with the use of nutritional supplements, adopting an anti-inflammatory/hypo-allergenic diet, and improving Gastrointestinal function. Eating healthy, regular bowel movements and lactobacillus supplementation can help with this.
- *Safe living environment:* Eliminate substances such as parabens (in cosmetics), phthalates (in pliable plastics), Bisphenol A (in plastics), PCBs and PBDEs (in coolants, flame retardants). Not only do these toxins produce similar side effects like the reproductive hormones of the body, they are linked to both infertility and cancer.
- *Lowering stress*: Chronic stress is linked to both hormonal disruption and inflammation. Relaxing and limiting stress is important to re-establish hormonal balance.
- *Yoga and Pilates:* Find activities you enjoy such as walking, swimming and yoga/Pilates. In contrast to high-intensity activities like running, spinning and

impact aerobics, yoga boosts blood flow into the internal organs by releasing tightness in the muscles of the hips, groin and lower back.

Treating Infertility

There are different ways to treat infertility.

Drugs: Various fertility drugs may be used for women with ovulation problems. It is important to talk with your doctor about the drug to be used. You should understand the drug's benefits and side effects. Depending on the type of fertility drug and the dosage prescribed, multiple births (such as twins) can occur. You should be prepared for that.

Surgery: Surgery is done to repair damage to a woman's ovaries, fallopian tubes or uterus. For a man, infertility problems that can be corrected by surgery include varicocoele and issues in the vas or sperm duct.

Intrauterine insemination (IUI): Also called artificial insemination. Male sperm is injected into part of the woman's reproductive tract, such as into the uterus or fallopian tube. IUI is often used along with drugs that cause a woman to ovulate. The sperm can be the partner's or donor sperm.

Assisted Reproductive Technology (ART): There are still many cases wherein conception is not possible with all this assistance. In such instances, fertilization of the egg with the sperm has to happen outside the body and this is known as In-vitro Fertilisation or IVF. Before fertilization, both the eggs and the sperm may need help, so a more holistic phrase for the same is Assisted Reproductive Technology or ART.

There is new technique where as part of IVF the sperm can be directly injected into the egg, but it is an advanced procedure. The idea is to optimize the chances of union and then sustain the growth of the embryo.

ART involves multiple steps which can be listed as follows:

- Stimulating a woman's ovaries to produce more and better quality eggs.
- Removing the eggs from her body.
- Mixing them with sperm in the laboratory.
- Putting the embryos back into the woman's body.

Success rates of ART vary and depend on many factors including skill of the specialist, motivation of the patient and emotional counselling apart from the health and medical reasons listed earlier in the chapter.

Third party assistance: Third part assistance include some of the following:

- Donor eggs (eggs from another woman are used).
- Donor sperm (sperm from another man are used).
- Surrogacy (when another woman carries a baby for you).

Finding the cause of infertility is often a long, complex and emotional process, and treatment can be expensive. It is important to undergo couple counselling, understand the chances of conception and the emotional trauma that is involved so one can be fully prepared to last the course. Many couples require multiple rounds of IVF for success and the process can be physically and emotionally taxing. Family support and hand-holding are vital to keeping couples motivated.

Quick tips for couples treating infertility:

1. Accept the trauma of trying to conceive.
2. Work on it with your partner equally.
3. Understand that the process could be long and taxing.
4. Discuss how far both of you are willing to go.
5. Discuss how much you are willing to pay for treatments/ procedures.
6. Educate yourself adequately.
7. Be prepared for the possibility of multiple births.
8. Be prepared for failure but be optimistic.
9. Relax do not let the process overpower you.
10. Talk about your misgivings with a friend, relative or counsellor.

TO SUMMARIZE

Infertility could be in the men or women

In women, chances for conceiving decrease after 35

Assess your situation with tests, hormonal profile, USG

Choosing correct time is critical

Options include oral medications, surgery, ART including IVF

Emotional counselling critical

9

Low Blow

Sunitha is a dear friend of mine. She is 46, bubbly, has a high-powered job and is the mother of an 18-year-old girl who has just gone off to university a few months ago. Off late, I have found that Sunitha has become very withdrawn. She hardly ever calls and even when I do, sounds dispirited and listless. Her husband called me to tell me that she is tired all the time and does not even feel like going to work. She just gets into her nightie and prefers to stay in bed most of the time except for meal timings. He told me he is really worried about her.

I met Sunitha and tried to draw her out to find out what was bothering her. It was fairly clear to me that she was suffering from acute clinical depression. I convinced her to go see a psychologist friend of mine, who gently spoke to her and made her open up. His conclusion was that she was suffering from depression, possibly arising out of an 'empty nest syndrome' with her daughter just going away. Sunitha was also experiencing erratic periods with a lot of pre-menstrual symptoms, which were adding to the problem, so he referred her to a gynaecologist to assess her. She is a little better now, slowly learning to adjust to this new phase of her life.

Sunitha is not alone. Depression is fairly common in women, especially in the teens and mid-30s upwards. Depression is defined as a mood disorder that manifests as lowered mood, loss of interest or pleasure, feelings of guilt or low self-worth, disturbed sleep or appetite, low energy and poor concentration.

Clinically, the feelings of sadness, hopelessness, helplessness and worthlessness occur when the brain produces an inadequate amount of serotonin, which is the chemical responsible for the regulation of mood. Depression is a serious condition that can impact your social life, relationships, career and sense of self-worth and purpose. And for women, in particular, depression is common. Roughly about one in eight women will develop depression at some point in her life.

Signs and symptoms of depression:

- Lowered mood.
- Loss of interest or pleasure in activities you used to enjoy.
- Feelings of guilt, hopelessness and worthlessness.
- Suicidal thoughts or recurrent thoughts of death.
- Sleep disturbance (sleeping more or sleeping less).
- Appetite and weight changes.
- Difficulty concentrating.
- Lack of energy and fatigue.

Women are about twice as likely as men to suffer from depression. The many causal factors include:

Biological and Hormonal Causes of Depression

Biology is a major reason for depression in a significant number of women. Many of these often remain unidentified and undiagnosed, therefore they tend to lie beneath the surface. The symptoms are usually noticed by a loved one, a co-worker or an acquaintance and then brought to the attention of the sufferer.

Pre-menstrual problems: Hormonal fluctuations can cause the familiar symptoms of pre-menstrual syndrome (PMS) such as bloating, irritability, fatigue and emotional reactivity. For many women, PMS is mild. But for some, symptoms are severe enough to disrupt their lives and a diagnosis of Pre-menstrual Dysphoric Disorder (PMDD) is necessary.

Pregnancy and infertility: The many hormonal changes that occur during pregnancy can contribute to depression, particularly in women already at high risk. Other issues relating to pregnancy such as miscarriage, unwanted pregnancy and infertility can also play a role in depression.

Post-partum depression: Many new mothers experience 'baby blues.' This is a normal reaction that tends to subside within a few weeks. However, some women experience severe, lasting depression, which is referred to as post-partum depression. Post-partum depression is believed to be influenced, at least in part, by hormonal fluctuations.

Peri-menopause and menopause: Women may be at increased risk of depression during peri-menopause, the stage leading to menopause when reproductive hormones fluctuate rapidly.

Women with past histories are at an increased risk of depression during menopause as well.

Health problems: Chronic illness, injury or disability can lead to depression in women, as can crash dieting or quitting smoking.

Psychological and Social Causes of Depression

Focusing on and rehashing negative feelings: Women are more likely to brood and rehash negative thoughts when depressed. This includes crying to relieve emotional tension, trying to figure out why you're depressed, and talking to your friends about your depression. However, this kind of continuous contemplation has been found to maintain depression and even make it worse. Men, on the other hand, tend to distract themselves when they are depressed. While it is catharitic to express negativity, it is important to not constantly dwell on it. Unlike contemplation, distraction can reduce depression.

Overwhelming stress at work, school or home: Some studies show that women are more likely than men to develop depression from stress and react more sharply to it. Women produce more stress hormones than men do, and the female sex hormone progesterone prevents the stress hormone system from turning itself off as it does in men.

Body image issues: The gender difference in depression begins in adolescence. This body dissatisfaction is perpetuated by the constant societal pressure on women to be sharply self-critical, resulting in depression.

Seasonal affect depression: Women in cold places develop

low feelings, believed to be due to the grey weather and lack of sunlight. This can affect men too.

Empty Nest Syndrome: When children grow up and leave home, some mothers experience a big void tinged with feelings of abandonment and worthlessness. This can lead to severe depression.

Treatments for Depression

Treatment of depression involves self-help, psychotherapy, counselling and medications.

Self-help: Self-help comprises helping oneself and asking for help from one's close relatives and friends. Some of the self-help measures that could help are:

- Talking about what makes you sad and expressing your feelings, within limits without letting the feelings overpower you.
- Doing activities that make you happy like watching a movie or meeting your parents.
- Writing your feelings down in a journal and not dwelling on them.
- Socializing, even when you don't feel like it.
- Joining a yoga class or learning meditation.
- Volunteering at a shelter or school. Looking after others can help you distract yourself from your problems.

In the case of hormonal depression, there are some measures which when adopted have been known to help women with depression significantly.

Exercise: Regular aerobic exercise can reduce the symptoms of hormonal depression. Exercise releases serotonin or the 'happy hormone'.

Dietary modifications: Changes to your diet may help reduce symptoms. Cutting back on salt, fatty foods, caffeine and alcohol is recommended. Eating plenty of complex carbohydrates like millet, oats and amaranth is also recommended.

Nutritional supplements: Vitamin-B6, calcium, magnesium, Vitamin-E, Omega-3 and Omega-6 and tryptophan have all been shown to benefit women suffering from PMDD.

Herbal remedies: Evening primrose oil and chaste tree berry are herbal supplements that have both been studied and found to be effective in the treatment of hormone-induced depression.

Stress reduction: Relaxation techniques and other strategies to reduce stress may help with hormonal symptoms. Yoga and meditation are particularly effective.

Counselling is critical in all stages of depression. When talking out things to closed ones does not help overcome the feelings of helplessness, it is wise to seek professional help and counselling. A few sessions with a professional have been proven to reverse depression very effectively.

There are various approved medications available for severe cases of depression. All of them must be administered under a psychiatrist's supervision. However, it must be kept in mind that even on medication, behavioural changes and counselling are vital to achieve long-term cures.

Most anti-depressants broadly aim to increase the levels of mood elevators like serotonin and norepinephrine. There are different types of anti-depressants like serotonin-specific reuptake inhibitors (SSRIs), tricyclic anti-depressants and monoamine oxidase inhibitors (MAOIs) that may be prescribed for different conditions depending on the severity of the depression. All of them must be prescribed, administered and supervised by a psychiatrist only.

Remember that depression is a common, often under-recognized and debilitating problem, in women. If you yourself or anyone you are close to is experiencing it, seek help immediately. Sometimes a shoulder to cry on can make all the difference between sadness, which you can get over, and clinical depression, which is more complex and long term.

TO SUMMARIZE

Depression can be debilitating

Family history is important

Find a good doctor to talk to

Medication, therapy critical

Support groups, family support make all the difference

10

Zit Fits, Razor Blades and the H Invasion

All of us know this feeling. There's an important presentation tomorrow; you go to sleep after carefully washing your face and applying night cream. In the morning you wake up with an uneasy feeling, look in the mirror and oh no, a big fat pimple, right in the middle of the chin—literally overnight!

When you look closer to examine the pimple, you notice three stubby, coarse, dark hairs sticking out of the chin. Oh my God, this cannot happen to me! Pimples, facial hair—what did I do wrong?

And then you call a friend and explain in a half sob what the issue is. She says, 'Don't worry. It's your hormones...'

Rather than being reassuring, this statement sets off another panic reaction. *Hormones?* What does that mean? Am I menopausal? Is this going to happen all the time? What do I do?

Well, the first thing to do is to breathe deeply and relax. Hormones are not per se our enemies. They are actually important for creating harmony in the body. Hormones are chemical messengers that transfer information and instructions from one set of cells to another. Controlled by a master computer called the endocrine system, hormones regulate every cell and function in our bodies. At any given time, the endocrine system releases more than 20 kinds of hormones into the bloodstream, where they can exert their influence on the specific body part they were designed for. Organs such as the pancreas, brains, heart, lungs, kidneys, liver, skin and placenta also secrete hormones.

How Do Hormones Affect the Skin?

Hormones can affect the skin in a number of ways. For most women, the introduction to imbalanced skin begins in adolescence with pimples, spots and excessive oiliness often accompanying the body's first hormonal peak. While for many the temperamental skin of our teen years fades with age, for others it is a concern that continues well into adulthood. Even for those with relatively well-balanced skin, intermittent fluctuations—such as during menstruation, starting or stopping birth control or the onset of menopause—can wreak havoc on one's complexion, particularly in terms of moisture balance.

Hormones affect moisture balance by stimulating the skin's sebaceous glands—natural, oil-producing glands—to produce more or less sebum, or natural oil, than normal. Elevated levels of the male hormone testosterone (yes, we women too secrete it!), for instance, tend to encourage sebum overproduction, often leading to an oily, blemish-prone complexion. Decreased levels of the female hormone oestrogen, on the other hand, result in drier skin as sebum production is scaled back.

Sebum production, however, is not the only factor influenced by the body's internal chemistry. Recent scientific evidence suggests a strong link between oestrogen and collagen production, with elevated levels of the hormone playing a key role in stimulating production of the structural tissue. Low hormone levels lead to dryness, wrinkles, sallow skin—all signs of skin ageing. Overactive hormones, on the other hand, make the skin oily, thick and prone to acne.

Acne

One of the main reasons for acne is the overactive action of hormones known as androgens, which include testosterone, DHEAS (a precursor of testosterone) and others. Yes, women have testosterone too, although in much smaller amounts compared to men. Testosterone stimulates the sebaceous glands, causing an excessive production of oil. The pores get plugged up, trapping bacteria from the environment. When the immune system detects the presence of the bacteria, it sets off an immune response in the skin, causing redness, swelling, pus, and eventually scarring if not treated well.

Testosterone levels tend to increase a week before your period, hence the acne during the pre-menstrual stress period, especially in your late 30s and 40s.

Although acne is the most commonplace symptom, there are other effects of hormonal stress on the skin. Some of these are:

Wrinkles and fine lines

As you age, oestrogen production in the ovaries decreases, which also accounts for reduced fertility over time. Oestrogen is also known as the 'female hormone' because it is responsible for almost all feminine characteristics such as clear skin, a shapely figure, and bone and heart health.

Oestrogen is also responsible for the production of hyaluronic acid, collagen and elastin, the very substances in costly anti-ageing beauty products. After the age of 40, oestrogen levels begin dipping and the skin starts to lose its elasticity. That is why you begin to see fine lines and wrinkles usually beginning around the eyes.

Interestingly, oestrogen is stored in fat, so excessively thin people tend to age faster. Watch your diet, but keep a healthy balance!

Dry, sagging skin

Dry skin is also the effect of decreased oestrogen. It can also happen with hypothyroidism, where you are low on the thyroid hormones produced by the thyroid gland located at the front of your throat. Low thyroid function makes the skin dry and scaly. Other symptoms of hypothyroidism are fatigue, muscle weakness, depression, joint pains and sensitivity to cold. Most women who are going through a low thyroid phrase describe themselves as 'feeling and looking lousy'.

Hyper-pigmentation (melasma)

Melasma are brown patches of skin that occur when oestrogen and progesterone produce more melanin pigments when exposed to the sun. Areas such as the forehead, nose and cheeks are common target areas.

Studies show that genetic factors play a part in determining whether you get melasma. Women with thyroid problems are more prone to melasma. Recent studies also suggest that chronic stress decreases cortisol, another vital hormone in the body, which in excess causes many skin problems and can bring about a melasma outbreak.

Melasma is a difficult condition to treat. The pigmentation, especially if it is deeper in the skin, is resistant to all kinds of topical treatments. Sun protection is a must to not allow the problem to worsen externally.

Rosacea

Rosacea, characterised by red, blotchy, itchy and flushed skin, is common among post-menopausal women. Oestrogen acts as an anti-inflammatory agent. When the body no longer produces sufficient oestrogen, it is more prone to skin inflammation. Rosacea usually appears on the face and can get worse with sun exposure. In severe cases, the entire face can appear strikingly red and sore.

For treatment of rosacea you need to consult a dermatologist. It is important to use mild cleansers and low dose topical antibiotic creams as well as soothing creams to treat the area.

Remember, your skin acts as a barrier to the rest of your body. It is also the first thing people notice about you, so consider investing in good skin to look and feel good inside-out!

Excessive facial hair (hirsutism)

Many women often find that they have started sprouting

coarse hairs on the chin, developing side burns and hairs on the moustache area. Around the same time, spots start appearing on the skin. The hair is really stubborn and reappears quickly after threading or waxing. Many women have shared with me how they have resorted to shaving their chins every single day to avoid the unseemly appearance of thick bristly hair that appears without fail in a day or two. Some causes of excessive facial hair may be use of Corticosteroids (oral and topical), obesity and PCOS.

So does everyone suffer from one or the other problem in their 30s and 40s?

Every single woman will usually experience some of these manifestations of hormonal play at some point in her thirties and forties. However, there are certain medical conditions that make women more prone to these symptoms.

Polycystic Ovary Syndrome (PCOS)

Women with PCOS often have hirsutism in combination with acne, balding near the front of the head, and menstrual irregularities. PCOS is also associated with other medical problems such as infertility (due to irregular menstrual cycle), obesity, diabetes mellitus, high cholesterol levels and possible heart disease.

PCOS is caused by hormonal imbalance. This imbalance promotes the unusual hair growth and may cause women to have unusually high levels of testosterone as well. The high level of testosterone causes the acne, hair growth and receding hairline. This imbalance can also block egg growth and inhibit ovulation.

Cushing's Syndrome

Cushing's Syndrome, a condition caused by having too much cortisol in the bloodstream, also causes excessive facial hair. Cushing's Syndrome may be caused by a tumour in the body as well, which should be treated through surgery and radiation. This condition might also be a side effect of Corticosteroid medications. Other symptoms of this condition are headaches, bruising, weight gain and fatigue.

Obesity

Women who are overweight may see an increase in facial hair. Fat traps androgens, creating hormonal imbalance. Because weight gain, adult acne and facial hair are signs of other conditions and disorders, women should go through a thorough medical examination to ascertain that there are no other underlying issues. Along with other physical characteristics, ancestry and genetics play a role in whether a woman will have facial hair. If your grandmother and mother had to pluck their chins and pop their zits or pimples, chances are you will, too.

Treatments

Hormonal Acne

For acne closely related to your period, you may need to do something hormonally to intervene. It may require the combined advice of a dermatologist, gynaecologist and an endocrinologist. Treatment options are multiple and may include the following:

Birth control pills

Birth control pills may help women who see a clear link between their acne and periods. Anything that raises oestrogen levels will lessen the effects of testosterone in women. Birth control pills work by increasing a protein called Sex-Hormone Binding Globulin (SHBG) in the blood. SHBG acts like a sponge, soaking up the free testosterone in the bloodstream. This means there is less testosterone available to cause acne.

Birth control pills also work by slowing down oil production. A combination of Ethinyl Estradiol with Cyproterone acetate is as effective and has fewer side effects than progesterone-containing pills.

If you start using birth control pills to control acne, be patient. When some women begin taking the pill, they experience an increased outbreak of acne for the first three to four months in response to the change in hormones. This should subside as your body adjusts to the new rhythm.

The biggest quandary in the treatment of hormonal acne with birth control pills is determining the end point of treatment. It is usually empirical and decided by the doctor depending on the patient response. Some women may experience bloating, dryness and even giddiness when using oral contraceptive pills. If you get any of these symptoms, inform your doctor immediately.

Spironolactone

If the acne doesn't respond to birth control pills alone, your doctor may add medication to lower your testosterone levels. This medication, called Spironolactone, curbs testosterone-related oil production in the skin. Side effects include breast tenderness, irregular periods, headaches and fatigue. Spironolactone is not appropriate for all women so do discuss its risks and benefits with your doctor.

Diet and skin care

A healthy diet plays a big role in adult acne. Sugar and milk have been found to cause acne in adult women, so cutting down both helps. Ensure you eat sufficient quantities of other foods rich in calcium. Include more protein and red- and orange-coloured fruits and vegetables in your diet to ensure inflammatory levels are down.

The basics of skin care include:

- Wash your face twice a day with a mild, perfume-free cleanser.
- Avoid touching your face; your hands introduce dirt and bacteria.
- Clean your cell phone regularly; phones are the breeding ground for a lot of bacteria, and you hold them against the area most vulnerable to hormonal acne: your jawline and chin.
- When you work out at the gym, cover all mats with a towel; don't put your face in other people's germs.
- Don't smoke; smoking is a contributory factor to all types of acne.
- Use tea tree oil containing cleansers.

For adult acne that is more severe, see a dermatologist who can prescribe medications like Isotretinoin, which is a natural derivative of Vitamin-A. The drug comes with a number of side effects and potential drug associations, especially birth defects in pregnant women; discuss all these risks with your doctor before using it.

If you have deep-seated pimples, your doctor may recommend oral and topical medications. A dermatologist can ease menstrual acne by performing some in-office treatments. Treatments may include cortisone injections, acne surgery, laser therapy, or a chemical peel.

Topical antibiotics, Benzoyl Peroxide and topical Retinoid may help but mostly as adjuvant treatments.

Treatment of hirsutism

Treatment of hirsutism, in addition to hormonal medications, verges on removal of hair through various temporary and semi-permanent methods. I'm going to give a very brief overview of some of these methods.

Shaving is the simplest and most widely used technique for removing hair. While most women use it on larger body parts, some women also use it for stubborn chin hair. The hair seems to come back faster because hair is cut more superficially than in other hair removal methods. Shaving on the reverse can promote ingrowing hairs and coarse stubble which may be socially stigmatizing.

Electrolysis, a method in which hair roots are destroyed by subjecting them to electric pulses, is a permanent method of hair removal. Electrolysis can be painful and the entire process takes multiple sessions and several months.

Threading is perhaps the most commonly used method of getting rid of unwanted facial hair. In this method thread is used to remove the hair from its roots. The only drawback of this method is that its effects are not long-lasting and so has to be repeated every other week.

Waxing the hair on the upper lip as well as on the side of the cheeks can help get rid of them for at least three weeks. Like threading, this method has to be repeated again and again as it is temporary.

Laser hair removal, in which the skin with unwanted hair is passed through laser beams which destroy the dark pigments in facial hair through the heat generated by the beams, can remove unwanted hair for about two to three years. Laser sessions need to be multiple at monthly intervals for about four to six sessions continuously after which multiple maintenance sessions may be needed.

Creams: Eflornithine Hydrochloride (Vaniqua) is a skin cream that can be used to slow the growth of unwanted facial hair in women. It does not remove hair permanently. Noticeable results take about six to eight weeks, and once the cream is discontinued, hair returns to pre-treatment levels after about eight weeks.

The other problems due to hormonal imbalance like melasma need the intervention of a dermatologist. A regular skin care routine and a healthy diet cannot be overemphasised in terms of their importance in the treatment of these conditions. Small changes in lifestyle can pay big dividends in the way your skin looks and behaves for the better.

A final word: It is often said jokingly that women are

moody because they have pre, intra or post-menstrual symptoms or menopause. It is indisputable that hormones do affect our moods and emotions and make us more vulnerable and labile. But it is also true that positive energy and emotions can influence hormone secretion in the body as can regular sleep habits. Both affect the normal cycles and rhythms in the body known as circadian rhythms. So the old adage of 'early to bed, early to rise, a proper diet and laughter in our lives' can definitely help us achieve harmony with our bodies and our hormones.

TO SUMMARIZE

Acne, hair loss can be severe and pigmentation common

Visit a dermatologist if symptoms are severe

Use a sunscreen when stepping out

Medication may be oral or topical or both

Hair growth on some areas may warrant removal

11

Oops! I Peed in My Pants

All of us have had that moment! That moment when we are watching an incredibly funny episode of *Friends* or are plagued with a sudden bout of intense coughing when, suddenly, a few warm drops trickle into our panties, followed by a few moments of truly crippling mortification. When it happens for the first time, it feels like that moment of truth, that moment when we realize that getting older is here, when we lose control of something important in the body, and this is a completely sobering experience.

To just reassure fellow tricklers, a little involuntary peeing is completely natural and nothing to press alarm bells about. However, if you notice it happening a little more frequently, it is important to find out the reason and what can really be done to prevent and/or correct it.

So What Is Involuntary Peeing?

Peeing without voluntary control is medically called urinary incontinence. The kind of involuntary incontinence we are talking about is known as Stress Urinary Incontinence or

SUI. Although there are various underlying causes for this condition, the fundamental issue is that of weakness in the pelvic muscles in women. Most cases of stress incontinence are due to weakened pelvic floor muscles, often weakened by childbirth.

The pelvic floor muscles are a group of muscles wrapped around the underside of the bladder and rectum. Stress incontinence is common in women who have had children, particularly if they have had several vaginal deliveries.

It is also more common with increasing age as the muscles become weaker, particularly after menopause. Being overweight with a poor muscle tone overall can also add to the problem. In a small percentage of women it can occur during regular menstruation as well.

So whatever the underlying cause, the mechanism of trickling pee without control is the same. The muscles in the pelvis weaken one way or the other, either temporarily or permanently. This can cause the bladder to drop down to a position that prevents the urethra from closing completely. The result is a leakage of urine when there is an increase in the pressure inside the abdomen. When we look at remedies, we need to consider both what causes the pelvic muscles to weaken and what causes the pressure in the abdomen to go up.

To hold urine and control urination, the lower urinary tract and nervous system need to be working normally. One must also be able to recognize and respond to the urge to urinate.

The average adult bladder can hold over two cups (350-550 ml) of urine. Two muscles are involved in controlling urine flow:

- The sphincter, which is a circle-shaped muscle around the urethra. You must be able to squeeze this muscle to prevent urine from leaking out.
- The detrusor, which is the muscle of the bladder wall. This must stay relaxed so that the bladder can expand.

In stress incontinence, the sphincter pelvic muscles, which support the bladder and urethra, are weakened. The sphincter is not able to prevent urine from flowing when pressure is placed on the abdomen (such as when you cough, laugh, or lift something heavy).

Stress incontinence may occur from weakened pelvic muscles that support the bladder and urethra or because the urethral sphincter is not working correctly.

What causes our pelvic muscles to weaken?

- Ageing and genetic factors: Ageing tends to worsen all forms of muscular injury. Changes in pelvic muscles can contribute to urinary incontinence.
- Multiple vaginal deliveries, especially after the age of 30.
- Previous pelvic surgery like uterine prolapse surgery or hysterectomy (uterus removal).
- Infections and medications: Urinary tract infections can cause temporary incontinence, and certain medications like sleeping pills and muscle relaxants may increase the likelihood of temporary incontinence.
- Obesity can worsen pelvic and abdominal muscle tone.
- Alcohol in excess also weakens the strength of the bladder.
- Repeated urinary tract infections can lead to weakening bladder muscles in women.

- Medical and neurological conditions such as hysterectomies, spinal problems, multiple sclerosis and Parkinson's disease can aggravate urinary incontinence.

How to Diagnose SUI?

You must think what a silly question this is! If I am peeing in my pants, I will obviously know. But, sometimes, it is not so simple. A little bit of peeing can happen to anyone anytime: when you are laughing very hard, or you have a sudden bout of violent coughing, or you haven't gone to the rest room for a long time. For you to suspect SUI, small triggers should repeatedly cause leakages, so do not press the panic button the moment you read this.

What you really need to watch out for is this: How often do you involuntarily leak a little bit? Do you feel there are times when you do not even have the urge to pee but you still leak a bit of urine? And does this leakage coincide with laughing, coughing, lifting weights or climbing the stairs? If your answer is yes to any of these questions, then indeed it is time for you to see a doctor.

The diagnosis of SUI is largely based on history, which means whatever you tell the doctor will help him or her make a definitive diagnosis. However, the doctor may ask you some probing questions to help make the final diagnosis. Some of the leading questions will be:

- How often do you leak urine?
- When you leak urine, is it a few drops or do your clothes get soaked?
- How often do you urinate in the toilet during the day and how often do you wake up at night?

- Do you drink beverages with caffeine or alcohol? How many each day?
- Do you drink a lot of fluids after 6 p.m.?
- What bothers you the most about your incontinence?

The major problem that women face with SUI is embarrassment, both personal and social. A patient of mine actually told me that she hated going out of her house for she always felt like she smelt of pee. So rule number one is: do not hide but seek help. You can make it better, but first go see a doctor!

Tests to Detect SUI

While very often history alone is enough to make a diagnosis, there are occasions when a doctor will ask for a few tests to corroborate the same. Some of these are:

- A urine sample to test for infection, traces of blood or other abnormalities.
- A neurological exam to identify sensory problems.
- A urinary stress test in which the doctor observes urine loss when you cough or bear down.
- A pad test.
- An Electromyogram to study muscle activity in the urethra or pelvic floor.
- Pelvic Ultrasound with a full bladder and then with the bladder emptied to check if there is complete voiding.

A simple test for diagnosis is the not-often-used pad test. The doctor asks you to wear a pad which has been dry weighed. You will then be asked to do ten minutes of vigorous exercise.

The pad is weighed again afterwards to check if it has gained weight due to incontinent voiding during exercise.

Treatment of SUI is not simple. It requires a multi-pronged approach to be truly effective—what I call BEST:

- B: Behavioural modification
- E: Exercise
- S: Stimulation
- T: Therapies

Behaviour Modifications

This is one of those conditions where simple behavioural modifications actually work. They are fairly easy to follow and pay rich dividends in terms of resolution of symptoms.

Decrease any excessive fluid intake

Okay, I am not telling you to stop drinking water. However, it is not wise for you to indulge in liquid diets, fad therapies like drinking three to four litres of water a day, etc. Continue drinking your normal quantity of water and try to space it out through the day so as not to put excessive pressure on the bladder at any given point in time.

Keep a pee diary

I know this sounds really funny, but this is sometimes the singlemost important intervention to help you with your diagnosis. Record every pee, the voluntary and the involuntary leakages, so you know the diagnosis for sure!

Pee more often

Urinating more frequently empties the bladder fully. It also ensures that there is no urine to leak in case of abdominal pressure.

Reduce high-impact exercises

Change your physical activities to avoid jumping or running movements, which can cause more urine leakage.

Regulate bowel movements

Constipation can worsen incontinence. Ensure enough fibre in your diet to avoid that.

Quit smoking

It will reduce coughing and bladder irritation.

Avoid alcohol and caffeine

Both of these overstimulate the bladder.

Avoid food and drinks that irritate the bladder

Spicy foods, carbonated beverages and citrus fruits—all irritate the bladder.

Lose weight and keep blood sugar under control

Both these help by reducing intra-abdominal pressure on the bladder.

Exercise

Here we are talking about a specific kind of exercise known as Kegel's.

Dr Arnold Kegel was an American gynaecologist who first described the benefits of Kegel's exercises in 1948. This is a very simple exercise which is extremely effective and is now recommended as a first line of therapy for SUI. It can be done any time, anywhere, sitting, standing or lying down. I will simplify the steps here:

- Empty your bladder.
- Find a comfortable position; for beginners I recommend lying down.
- Focus your mind on your lower pelvic region.
- Contract the muscles in your pelvic area without contracting your tummy muscles. Your action will be similar to the action you do to hold in your pee.
- In case you cannot understand lower pelvic area, insert a finger in your vagina and try and contract the muscles around your finger.
- Hold in the contracted position for a minute building up to three.
- Relax for a minute and then repeat.
- You can do ten repetitions five to six times a day.

Some women have a little trouble getting started with Kegel's. Talk to your gynaecologist. Vaginal cones may be recommended to be inserted inside your vagina to provide some weight and indication as to the correct technique of Kegel's. Bio feedback techniques using simple monitors to ensure you are doing your procedure properly are also very useful. These are simple measurement techniques linked to the exercises which can give you feedback on how effective they are.

Yoga

There are certain yoga asanas which too help in controlling incontinence. I recommend that you do these only under the expert guidance of a trained yoga teacher. These are:

- Dronasana or boat pose
- Sethu bandhasana or bridge pose
- Mula bandha or core stop technique

Exercise alone can reverse and help maintain bladder control in most sufferers of SUI. Needless to say, regularity of the exercise is the most important factor to sustain long-term results.

Electrical Stimulation

The effectiveness of this procedure is oft debated but seems to help in those women who find it hard to do Kegel's properly. In this method, electrodes are temporarily inserted into your rectum or vagina to stimulate and strengthen the pelvic floor muscles.

This is usually done as an outpatient procedure but nowadays home care units are also available. A tampon-like sensor that connects to a handheld adjustable device is inserted in the vagina.

Gentle electrical stimulation can be effective for stress

incontinence and urge incontinence, but it takes several months and multiple treatments to work. Units are available for home usage as well and can be used after checking with your doctor.

Therapies

Various therapies, both non-surgical and surgical, have been known to control stress urinary incontinence. Some of them are:

Collagen injections

Collagen injections given into the lining of the urethra or the neck of the bladder act as bulking agents by either bringing the walls of the urethra closer together or sealing off the base of the bladder. This allows the urethra to close tightly enough to prevent urine from leaking out. The result is similar to the way the body functions naturally and, in most cases, urinary control will be improved and restored. If a patient is allergic to collagen, other bulking agents or fillers are also available.

Taping procedures

Simple outpatient minor surgeries taping the vagina tighter are sometimes done when other measures listed above do not work well. This is required especially in those women where there may be a mild vaginal prolapse following multiple vaginal deliveries.

The purpose of all these taping procedures is to provide support under the urethra to ensure that it closes properly, preventing leakage of urine involuntarily.

Sling Surgeries

The purpose of sling surgeries is to support a weak bladder by providing support to it through simple slings or muscular supports. Sling surgeries can be performed as an outpatient procedure and nowadays are done laparoscopically.

SUI is not a condition to get you upset or shed tears over! It is so eminently possible to control it through your own efforts, so take that first step to identify and accept that it is happening to you. Once this is done, the BEST approach can be employed early enough to arrest it and improve your quality of life.

TO SUMMARIZE

SUI

- What is it?

  Involuntary leakage of urine
- Who gets it?

  Overweight, multiple pregnancy, post-35 women
- Diagnosis: Clinical

  Rule out infections of bladder
- Treatment

  BEST Approach: Behaviour, Exercise, Stimulation, Therapies

12

Scalp that Hair

There is a moment of truth for every woman. To me, it was looking at my face while brushing my teeth in a hotel bathroom with bright yellow lights. I suddenly noticed a patch in the front of my scalp. I looked closer and realized my entire crown had the skin underneath the hair visible and I promptly burst into tears.

Next to acute Telogen Effluvium, Female Pattern Hair Loss or FPHL is the second-most common cause of diffuse hair loss in women. This is known commonly as female balding where the hair starts thinning from the top. FPHL causes tremendous psychological distress to women as it is age-related. Although it can be considered similar to male androgenic alopecia, there are a number of significant differences between the two, making prognosis and treatment of the condition different.

Age of occurrence

FPHL appears to have two different patterns of occurrence. The first, less common, one afflicts younger women in their late 20s and early 30s and has a definitive genetic and androgenic basis. The second kind appearing in women in their late 40s and early 50s is more age and senescence related but has a hereditary component usually present.

How do I know if I have FPHL?

The first and most common symptom of FPHL is widening of the parting area. A lot of women notice that in the frontal area of the head the hair appears to be getting more wispy and thin. It is also not uncommon to have the hair loss first noticed and commented upon by your hair stylist.

So what does one look out for?

There are some insidious signs that a lot of us ignore or are in denial about.

- ❑ Do you spend longer than usual arranging the front of your hair?
- ❑ Has someone taller than you commented on your scalp showing?
- ❑ Do you find yourself skipping the conditioner, especially the leave-in serum, on the top and front portion of your hair because it flattens your hair and makes it look thinner?
- ❑ Have you started buying volumizing shampoos?
- ❑ Do you avoid styling your hair with a parting?
- ❑ Have you switched to wider-toothed, softer combs recently?

Even if your answer is yes to just one of these questions, do think about seeing a dermatologist immediately!

What can a dermatologist do?

There are of course many things a dermatologist can and will do! The first is to note down your complete medical history and conduct a physical examination of your hair and scalp. One of the classic signs is the abovementioned widened parting at the top, front and back of the scalp (occiput) although the front margin itself may be reasonably well maintained. The hair is thinner, wispier and resembles the appearance of vellus hair which is thin hair found in certain parts of the body like the arms. Although different grades and patterns have been described, they are not as clear cut or well defined as male pattern hair loss and hence seeing a dermatologist early becomes important.

The dermatologist may recommend some tests to rule out increase in circulating androgens, polycystic ovarian disease and thyroid problems. However, a lot of the tests may actually come negative as even when the tests are normal, there is also a possibility of increased hormones only locally at the scalp. Some women also may have an increased scalp sensitivity to even normal circulating hormones so blood tests do not always provide the correct picture. Hormonal problems like PCOD are more commonly seen with early onset of FPHL. The role of 5 Alpha Reductase, so strong in male balding, is unclear with the response to both Finasteride and its newer cousin Dutasteride being neither impressive nor predictable. Hence, it can be assumed that younger women with other hormonal imbalance signs like weight gain and insulin resistance should definitely be considered for androgen sensitivity signs that warrant doing tests. The physician, however, will finally decide on the tests that you may need to do before starting treatment for this kind of hair loss.

Diagnosis

Diagnosis continues to be largely clinical supported only by various tests as described above. The dermatologist will first rule out possibilities like chronic Telogen Effluvium or shedding hair loss as opposed to hair thinning, starvation and FAD diets before making a diagnosis, doing investigative tests and starting treatment. Factors like anaemia and hypothyroidism will also be looked into before embarking on a treatment. A lot of dermatologists may use an instrument called the derma scope which gives characteristic images for different hair conditions.

Treatment Options

Topical applications

Treatment options are fairly limited for FPHL as opposed to MPHL (Male Pattern hair Loss), but early intervention can bring about good results. Each one of us reacts differently to the fact of hair loss and it is very important to share the extent of your distress with the dermatologist and to have it addressed in an empathetic and supportive fashion. This can sometimes play an extremely important role in getting the best outcomes from the medications.

To be effective the medications should ideally be able to do three things:

- Convert telogen hair (shedding) to anagen hair (growing).

- ❑ Delay the onset of catagen to make anagen longer.
- ❑ Try and ensure that a more mature, thicker, terminal hair is produced in anagen.

The one medication that is approved for safe use in female pattern hair loss is Minoxidil (two per cent). Minoxidil can be effective with the first two targets but, in terms of making the hair thicker, it can take a very long time. However, five per cent Minoxidil used by dermatologists in women has shown very good outcomes.

The ideal application of Minoxidil is twice daily and newer forms like foams and gels facilitate this dosage. Initially, on starting Minoxidil, it is common to experience some immediate hair loss due to discarded telogen hairs. Minoxidil must be used for at least six months before deciding on its efficacy and if stopped, hair loss will commence in three months.

But hey, it works! It has very few reported side effects other than irritation, usually due to the form in which it is applied rather than Minoxidil itself. It can rarely cause increased facial hair, hence care is advised especially during night application. It is best to remain in an upright position for at least 15-20 minutes after application and use less runny formulations like gels and foams.

Spironolactone cream is available on prescription in Western markets, but is yet to be launched in India.

Copper Peptides is another product available in Western markets that is believed to make the terminal hair stronger and thicker. It is available in shampoo/conditioner formats and is still to get complete approval from the USFDA.

Oral medications

The aim of oral medications in FPHL is to first fix underlying problems like anaemia and hypothyroidism and, second, to use anti-androgens to stimulate hair growth. Some of the options in the second category are oral Spironolactone, contraceptives with Cyproterone Acetate and 5 Alpha Reductase inhibitors.

Spironolactone inhibits production of testosterone and is useful in women with known androgen issues, especially excessive facial hair with scalp hair loss. But it can have significant side effects including electrolyte imbalance and must only be taken under strict and constant medical supervision.

Oral contraceptives

Oral contraceptives with Cyproterone Acetate have been used successfully in androgenic skin conditions like acne, excessive facial hair and scalp hair loss. Oral contraceptives with drospirenone are also effective. However, they have their own side effects and the end point of treatment is hard to determine, hence dermatologists use this option with great caution.

Surgical treatments

Hair transplants are done more frequently in women now, but suffice to say that in women results may only be modest at best and expectations need to be more realistic than in men.

Other modalities

Low-level lasers are gaining popularity in terms of being able to thicken the terminal hairs and stimulate dormant follicles to produce new hair. Simple measures like a very good haircut to camouflage observed thinning go a long way in keeping women motivated on treatments that take longer to produce results.

General measures

A balanced diet high in protein, iron and fibre is vital for good quality hair. Traditional Indian remedies like regular oil massages also help not only by increasing blood circulation to the follicles, but by true therapeutic benefits as discussed later. Stress-reducing measures like yoga, regular exercise and meditation also potentiate good outcomes.

The most important aspect to female pattern hair loss is the accompanying psychological trauma, so it is important find a good dermatologist, a good hair stylist and a good friend who can help you both laugh at the demonic proportions this simple condition can assume and to help you stay motivated on the treatments!

TO SUMMARIZE

Two types of hair loss: shedding and thinning

Nutrition is most important: protein, iron and biotin vital

Early treatment produces best results

Remedies are topical or oral, and may be a transplant

13

Going South and Raccoon Eyes

About nine months ago I got this email in my inbox. It was from a lady living in Jharkhand who was writing to me about her face. The words she used were these: 'Everything is getting coarse and loose. All my features seem to be getting less sharp, my skin is splotchy and I don't mind getting older, but I just feel so unattractive.'

The email set me thinking because this is what a lot of people tell me. It's not the age per se but the skin changes that alter one's perception of one's own attractiveness. But there is a way we can work towards preventing these obvious changes. We can work towards understanding our skin in the different decades and follow preventive measures to mitigate the ageing.

Tantalizing 30s

Okay, so you have hit the thirties and while you still feel like the belle of the ball, your skin has begun to show tell-tale signs of ageing. How can you identify these early signs and what steps can you take to counter them?

Eye Spy

The skin around the eyes is the most sensitive part of the facial skin. Early signs of ageing include fine lines, dryness of the skin and a dehydrated appearance.

What you can do: Use a special undereye cream with ingredients like Vitamin-K, Vitamin-C and Lactic acid with a mild sunscreen. Also buy a good lotion-based moisturiser to nourish the skin. Combine with a sunscreen during the day.

What you must eat: Beta Carotene containing anti-oxidants are very useful in combating early signs of ageing in this area. Get them naturally by eating fruits/veggies in the red-orange spectrum like carrots, pumpkin, beet root, etc.

A little more at the dermatologist's: Alpha Hydroxyl peels like Glycolic and Lactic peels can help build superficial collagen and reduce fine lines.

Pore Me Out

Enlargement of pores on the skin is one of the earliest signs of collagen loss and ageing. Typically seen on the cheeks and nose, this gives rise to an uneven bumpy appearance on the skin. This sign is often missed and needs special attention.

What you can do: Add an alcohol-free toner to your cleansing routine. Start using a prescription retinoid cream from a dermatologist, or retinol or an anti-oxidant cream with ingredients like Vitamin-E or Ubiquinone for night-time usage. Use a sunscreen religiously every single day.

What you must eat: Selenium and magnesium are potent preventive anti-ageing agents. They are found abundantly in whole grains like brown rice and millet. Make these a part of your diet.

A little more at the dermatologist's: Non-ablative photo rejuvenation using an Nd Yag laser along with a microdermabrasion works wonderfully to build collagen. Salicylic acid peels are also helpful.

Nosy Parker

Blackheads on the nose along with a special condition called trichostasis spinulosa leads to a dotted black appearance on the nose.

What you can do: Regular exfoliation using a Glycolic or Retinoic acid cream really helps in reducing this condition.

What you must eat: Vitamin-C aids in reducing the darkness and Vitamin-A in keratinization. Eat plenty of citric fruits and vegetables like carrots.

A little more: Hair removal on the nose combined with Salicylic peels can produce good results.

Fabulous 40s

The best decade for most women, it is also the time when you have to give your skin the attention it deserves. Some of the ageing signs to watch out for are:

Frown lines and crow's feet

Yup, all the expression in your life seem to settle on your

face. Lines when you raise your eyebrows, frown and smile are common and are known as dynamic lines of age.

The lower eyelid becomes a bit loose and crow's feet start fanning out from the corners of the eyes. This is known as cutaneous laxity.

What you can do: Relax your face. Practise yoga and meditation to relax the muscles on the face. Certain creams containing Argirilene can help diminish these lines. A great moisturizer is a must along with a sunscreen.

What you must eat: Maintain a constant healthy weight as weight loss will accelerate these lines. Include fibres like oats, vegetables and brown rice, whole grains and Omega-3 fatty acids in your diet.

A little more: A small injection of Botulinum toxin by an expert relaxes the muscles, making the lines vanish. It will need to be repeated every four months or so.

Laughter lines groove

The laughter lines or the naso-labial lines deepen and groove and become prominent on the lower third of the face.

What you can do: Use creams with a higher moisturizing power and special ingredients like Hyaluronic acid, Retinal, Alpha Lipoic acid and Vitamin-E and Collagen Peptides. Never miss your sunscreen or moisturizer even for a single day.

What you must eat: Fill your plate with colours. Eating multi-coloured foods will give you a great dose of anti-oxidants needed to keep the collagen busters at bay.

A little more at the dermatologist's: Collagen-based Hyaluronic acid temporary fillers can be injected to reduce the grooves. Minimally invasive lasers like Nd Yag and IPL (Intense Pulse Light) help to build collagen.

Melasma and pigmentation

Hormonal changes and sun exposure contribute to a mask-like pigmentation extending across the cheeks, nose and forehead.

What you can do: Niacinamide and Vitamin-C over-the-counter creams may help lighten the skin. For more severe cases prescription ingredients like Kojic acid, Arbutin and Hydroquinone may be needed.

A little more at the dermatologist's: Peels like Glycolic acid, TCA and yellow peels may be useful in individual cases. Pure Vitamin-C serum in topical form is also useful.

What you must eat: In the 40s, focus on your diet by including whole grains, pulses, coloured fruits and vegetables. All these aid in countering inflammation and reducing ageing. Decrease your intake of pro-inflammatory foods like simple sugars and saturated fats and watch yourself glow!

Feisty 50s

The changes that commence in the 40s tend to increase and deepen in the 50s. Hormonal changes also contribute to the visible ageing.

Sun spots, keratoses and skin tags

50s is the time of blotches and splotches. Continued sun exposure through the years tends to give rise to small, unseemly growths called keratoses, skin tags and lentigenes. These show up as growths on the face and neck.

What can you do: Regular use of sunscreens can prevent these.

A little more: Removal using radiofrequency machines or lasers is instantaneous and very effective.

Inflammatory changes and rosacea

The skin tends to get a blush and flush appearance due to inflammatory changes in the lymphatic system and blood vessels on the cheeks

What you can do: Stock up on Omega-3 fatty acids like fish, walnuts and olive oil to reduce inflammation. Focus on whole grains, fruits and vegetables.

Use anti-inflammatory products like aloe vera, ALA and calamine lotion to reduce the red. More severe rosacea will require a dermatologist's help. Hydrate your skin at all times by drinking enough water and use a moisturizer suited to your skin type.

What you must eat: Diet plays a key role in anti-aging. After 40, supplementation of vitamins and essential minerals can aid in preserving the skin's integrity. Get a good prescription anti-oxidant from your doctor, arm yourself with a sunscreen and face every age with renewed skin confidence.

Raccoon Eyes

Dark circles! Practically every single person I see has it, whether they seek help for it or not. It is very common in India; it is believed to be ethno-racial and have a strong genetic basis. Dark circles can range from mild darkening to severe raccoon eyes with rings of pigmentation. They are also often accompanied by puffiness, fine lines and wrinkles around the eyes which worsen their appearance even further.

Scientifically, dark circles are known as Peri-orbital Melanosis, which basically indicates a melanin mediated pigmentation in the undereye area. However, dark circles are also caused due to vascular reasons or inflammation arising out of the blood vessels and hence are one of the most difficult dermatological conditions to treat.

If you suffer from dark circles under your eyes, you're probably tired of people asking you if you're sick or tired, which can lower your self-esteem and make you hesitant to engage in social and work-related group activities.

What are the causes of dark circles?

Although there are plenty of reasons why one could get dark circles, there are some common reasons which may play a contributing role. Some of these are facial ageing, lifestyle causes and allergies of various natures.

Facial ageing and dark circles: Facial ageing and its early occurrence itself is genetic. It tends to cause volume loss from the cheeks and creates hollows in the undereye areas. This can actually lead to a hollowed-out appearance with sunken eyes like a crater. This, coupled with the volume loss of the thin undereye skin and the rupture of blood vessels, can cause the appearance of severe dark circles. The pouch of fat under the eye may, in addition, bulge out, making the dark circles even more prominent.

Genetic factors

- Volume loss or fat descent in the cheeks.
- Undereye volume loss.
- Lower eyelid (canthus) laxity.
- Thinning undereye skin.
- Bulging undereye fat.

Lifestyle choices and undereye circles

As we have seen in various chapters right through this book, lifestyle factors play a big role in causation of almost all health problems. It is also true in the case of dark circles. The top three factors are altered sleep habits, rubbing of the eyes constantly and smoking. Drinking a lot of alcohol and coffee also tend to promote undereye dark circles. One must watch out for poor dietary habits like not eating enough protein or vegetables, which may cause dietary deficiencies that promote dark circles.

One other common reason for dark circles is simply dehydration due to not drinking sufficient water. This can also be seen in fever conditions like viral fevers where the body experiences a state of dehydration that tend to give you dark circles.

Lifestyle factors

- Smoking
- Hyperpigmentation caused by sun damage
- Caffeine consumption
- Alcohol consumption
- Sleep deprivation
- Dehydration
- Other causes of eye circles

In addition to the main causes discussed above, there are some other causes of dark circles. These include nasal and sinusal allergies, hormonal pigmentation and venous fragility under the eyes, eczemas and seborrheic dermatitis amongst others. Very often, in these conditions, the dark circles diminish once the underlying condition is treated.

Other causes

- Hyperpigmentation caused by melasma
- Allergies
- Nasal congestion
- Medical conditions (eczema, thyroid problems, etc.)
- Venous congestion in under eye blood vessels
- Environmental exposure
- Heredity

Diagnosis of dark circles

Dark circles are almost always diagnosed by the patients themselves. The role of the doctor is to try to determine the underlying cause and offer appropriate treatments for the same. There is a way in which you can do a more informed self-diagnosis as well and I am going to teach you that little trick.

Look straight into a mirror in natural light, then lower your chin slightly to expose the shadows under your eyes. This way you'll see clearly whether your circles are bluer or browner.

Blue Circles

The cause: Blue circles result from oxygenated blood pooled beneath the undereye skin. The skin here is very thin and almost transparent, so blood shows through. This is more noticeable in the morning. When we've been lying horizontally for a while, fluids accumulate and the veins expand to hold more blood. Blue circles may get worse with age.

OTC treatments: There are a few options that work in different ways, though their effects last only a day at most. Topical creams with stimulating ingredients like caffeine can constrict blood vessels and temporarily boost circulation. Potent hydrators, such as Hyaluronic acid, plump the area, pushing the skin up and away from the pooled blood. Retinoic acid creams thicken the outer layer of the skin to conceal shadows

Quick fix: Use cold water compress. They constrict the blood vessels and cause instant improvement. A camouflage concealer can be applied right on top of it.

Professional treatments: One non-invasive solution is a cream with a prescription-strength retinoid. Blue circles can also be significantly diminished by a treatment called Thermage, which involves a high-tech handheld radio-frequency device. It is non-surgical, requires no downtime, and is thought to increase the production of collagen which builds up and tightens the skin. Nowadays, dark circles are also treated by injecting a Hyaluronic acid filler to plump the skin and hide blueness.

Brown Circles

Brown circles result from hyperpigmentation triggered by chronic eye-rubbing, sun exposure or genetics.

OTC treatments: Your best bet is daily use of a cream or serum spiked with a skin brightener, like soy or citrus, which can lighten circles over a period of four to six weeks. Kojic acid, Arbutin and Curcumin-containing creams are also a good bet in this area.

Professional treatments: As with blue circles, there are treatments dermatologists employ elsewhere on the face that can also lessen the look of brown circles. They respond well to low-concentration Glycolic, multi-ingredient lightening peel as well as judiciously employed TCA (Trichloroacetic Acid) peels which exfoliate the area.

Preventive measures

Prevention is indeed better and easier than cure when it comes to dark circles. Eat a healthy diet with plenty of fibre from oats, vegetables and fruits. Focus on eating adequate protein every day. Keep yourself rested and adequately hydrated. You can follow these steps:

- *Wear sunscreen*: It will keep circles from returning after treatment and can also stop them from developing in the first place. Sun protection prevents skin from both thinning prematurely (exposing blueness) and tanning (getting browner).
- *Wear large dark glasses*: Physical protection is the best sun protection.
- Sleep with a firm pillow to aid fluid drainage from the eye to facial lymphatics.
- Drink plenty of water to avoid dehydration.
- Sleep at least seven hours every night.
- Avoid rubbing and irritating the eyes.

Often dark circles require a cosmetic camouflage, especially for social reasons. For quick circle camouflage, apply eye cream and let it dry for a few minutes. Then pat on a creamy concealer that matches your skin tone. Top with a layer of loose powder.

Dark circles are one of the most vexing problems in dermatology. However, with adequate care and timely treatment, one can keep them under control and prevent them from marring the appearance of facial skin.

TO SUMMARIZE

Ageing has specific signs every decade

Preventive treatment in 30s, corrective treatment 40s upwards

Diet is critical: Anti-inflammatory foods like coloured fruits and vegetables

Dark circles are multi-factorial: Adequate sleep, right diet and simple care can be a huge preventive

Treatment ranges from medications to dermatological procedures to surgery

14

Back Up

'It began as a twinge, on days I had stood for too long. Then the pain started to radiate down my back when I walked on the treadmill. Yet I saw no reason to modify my fitness routine. I ran. I kick boxed. I lifted weights. And after about three weeks, I paid the price. One sleepless night, pain that felt like a knife in my back pinned me to the couch. I had to literally crawl my way out and be taken to a hospital. My disc had ruptured.'

This is the story of 41-year-old Rachita, but finds resonance with more people than I can count on my fingers.

And the ones who come to the surface comprise only the tip of the iceberg. So many more women experience twinges, aches and pains far more frequently than they let on. This is because so many activities we do every day cause stresses and strains on the backbone and the spine.

Everyday activities that you do without thinking—sitting at the computer, slipping on a pair of shoes, crawling into bed at night—can make or break your spine health. Most aches are caused by strains (injured muscles or tendons) or sprains (damage to the tough fibrous tissue, or ligaments, located where your vertebrae connect to joints). These injuries are typically brought on by over-use, a new activity, excessive lifting, a sudden jerk or an accident. Other times, a compressed (aka pinched) nerve, such as in a slipped disc, known medically as a herniated disk, is to blame for the ache.

Given the prevalence of back pain in women (close to 80 per cent), you would think we'd have readymade treatments for it. Not even close. The challenge is that you can't see injuries to tendons, ligaments and muscles the way you can perceive bone fractures and herniated disks. So despite diagnostic advances, doctors can't pinpoint the exact cause for as many as 85 per cent of back problems, which makes them tricky to treat.

If you fall into the 80 per cent of the population that regularly suffers from back pain, take heart: One-third of aches due to a strain or a sprain improve in a week without medical intervention (the remainder may take up to eight weeks). But unless you do some spine tuning and strengthening your back through exercise and fostering healthier habits, the odds of a recurrence within six months are about one in three.

Before we look at what can help the spine, we have to look at what causes maximum damage to the spine and how to avoid these bad habits.

Screen Preen

Nine hours is how long the average person spends hunched over or slouched in front of a screen each day. Couple this with smartphones and tablets and you have more aches than you can count on your shoulders, necks and backs. It's important to take breaks, do neck exercises, and occasionally hold your phone or tablet out in front of you, so you are not hunched over them all the time.

Tip

- For a simple neck reliever, hold your head for ten seconds in each of the following positions: forward, back, left and right. Repeat this five times a day.
- Take a break from sitting every one hour, walk around even if for a minute.

Get to the core

The general impression is that any talk of core means six pack abs and a sculpted body. But the core really supports the four pillars that strengthen the delicate spine. Back, side, pelvic, and buttock muscles all work together, along with your abs, to allow you to bend, twist, rotate and stand upright. The core is like a crane that supports all of one's movements. Unlike crunches, which focus solely on abdominal muscles, core exercises such as lunges, squats, planks strengthen several spine-supporting muscle groups at once.

Be like Goldilocks

Get a bed which is neither too hard nor too soft but is firm and just right. This is what actually supports the back best when you sleep. The ideal position to sleep is on your side or your back as this keeps your spine neutral and elongated. If you must snooze on your tummy, slide a thin pillow under your hips to alleviate pressure on disks, ligaments and muscles.

Lighten up

Controlled studies have proved that both acute and chronic stress can cause and worsen back pain. People with major depression are four times as likely to develop disabling lower back and neck pain. Some scientists believe that poor coping skills related to depression may trigger the release of the stress hormone cortisol, causing back and shoulder muscles to tense up and spasm resulting in chronic pain and depression which tend to be self-sustaining. Anti-depressants as well as mood enhancers like exercise, meditation, yoga and deep breathing can help ease stress and make you feel better.

But don't light up

Nicotine restricts blood flow to vertebrae and disks, so they may age and break down more quickly. It may also interfere with the body's ability to absorb and use calcium, leading to osteoporosis-related bone and back problems. The solution is single, if not simple: quit today and reap the benefits of a stronger back instantly

Heel and flat

Footwear plays a very big role in back pain. While we all know stilettos can cause joint pains, extremely flat footwear like sandals and flip flops also strain the back. Buy footwear with good arch support on the sides of the feet, and alternate styles through the week to relieve pressure on the spine.

Be moderately active

While too much strain is bad for the back, too much rest is

not good either. Low-impact activities like walking and swimming boost blood flow to the back muscles while relieving pain and stiffness. Yoga, with its emphasis on stretching and strengthening, may be one of the most effective spine soothers.

Self-care

Self-care plays a big role in early care and prevention of back pain.

- ❑ Moderate activity is most helpful, but avoid anything that makes the pain much worse. Staying in bed for more than two days can make back pain worse.
- ❑ Use ice or cold packs for twenty minutes three to four times a day during the first few days of a muscle sprain or spasm.
- ❑ A hot bath or heating pad can help reduce pain and stiffness. Use heat only after the first few days if you continue to experience pain.
- ❑ Take a medication for pain and inflammation. Pain killers like Ibuprofen and Naproxen help but do seek a doctor's advice.
- ❑ Maintain good posture to keep your body's weight aligned and reduce stress on the back muscles.
- ❑ Lying on your back with a pillow under your knees or lying on your side with a pillow between your lower legs can ease pain so you can sleep.
- ❑ Weight loss is important to prevent future problems.
- ❑ Return to work or your usual daily activities within a few days, with lighter duties or limited hours. This prevents your back from becoming weak and stiff.

- Avoid lifting heavy objects and repeated bending and twisting. Change positions often during the day and use a chair with good lower back support.
- Learn to accept and deal with stress. If you have some particular stress in your life, discuss it with your doctor.

Treatment

Muscle relaxers can be used during the first few days to ease muscle spasms, but they often cause drowsiness. In some instances, steroid medications may be injected directly into the epidural space (the space surrounding the nerves within the spinal canal) to ease sciatica pain. Physical therapy may be prescribed by your doctor if you have severe incapacitating pain for more than a week, no improvement after two weeks of home therapy, or if you are unable to return to work (or limited activity) within one week.

Prevention

Prevention is the most important tool for maintaining spine health.

- Good posture is important for keeping the spine healthy. Stand straight. Keeping your body aligned takes the stress off your back muscles.
- Avoid lifting heavy objects. When you do lift, bend your knees and keep your back straight.
- Maintain a healthy weight. If you are overweight, you will put more stress on your lower back.
- Try not to reach for objects that are above your head. Use a step stool or a device that helps you reach objects

on higher shelves. Store items that you use often on lower shelves.

- Avoid repeated bending or twisting.

Exercise and stretches for the back

- Yoga is a perfect exercise to strengthen the back.
- Pelvic tilt and pelvic bridging really help.
- Back stretches by lying flat on the back help too.

All exercise for the back must be learnt from a certified yoga teacher or physiotherapist. Remember that the back is sensitive and delicate and every single thing you do undermines its strength. A back-up plan to nurture the back is vital for a happy and healthy life.

In addition to protecting the spine, it is also necessary to build strong bones to ensure women are not plagued by aches and pains 30s upwards. In the next chapter, we will take a quick look at how to maintain and build bone strength.

TO SUMMARIZE

Back trouble can be chronic

Reasons would be bad posture, long hours of standing, strain and computer work

Preventive methods are anti-inflammatories, bed rest

Take calcium and Vitamin-D supplements, exercise moderately, do yoga or stretching

Lifestyle changes important

In extreme cases, surgery may be necessary

15

Handle with Care: Your Bones

Bones play many roles in the body: they provide structure, they protect the internal organs, they anchor the muscles and store calcium. While it's particularly important to take steps to build strong and healthy bones during childhood and adolescence, you can take precautions to protect bone health during adulthood too.

So why is bone health important?

Our bones are in a process of change throughout our lives. New bone is made and old bone gradually breaks down. When we are young, our body creates new bone quicker than it breaks down old bone, so our bone mass increases. Most people reach their peak bone mass at around the age of 30. After that, bone remodelling continues, but we begin to lose slightly more bone mass than we gain.

The likelihood of developing osteoporosis, a condition that causes bones to become weak and brittle, depends on one's bone mass as one touches 30 and the rapidity with which it is lost after that. The higher your peak bone mass, the more bone you have 'in the bank' and the less likely are you to develop osteoporosis as you age.

Factors Impacting Bone Health

Dietary calcium: A diet low in calcium contributes to diminished bone density, early bone loss and an increased risk of fractures.

Exercise: People who are physically inactive have a higher risk of osteoporosis than their more active counterparts.

Smoking/alcohol: Research suggests that tobacco use contributes to weak bones. Similarly, having more than two alcoholic drinks a day increases the risk of osteoporosis, possibly because alcohol can interfere with the body's ability to absorb calcium.

Gender: Women have lesser bone tissue than men, so they tend to develop osteoporosis sooner.

Weight: Extremely thin women and those with small body frames tend to have less bone mass which may become pronounced with age.

Hormone levels: Too much of the thyroid hormone can cause bone loss. In women bone loss increases dramatically at menopause due to the sharp fall in oestrogen levels. Prolonged periods and absence of menstruation (amenorrhea) before menopause also increases the risk of osteoporosis.

Medications: Long-term use of Corticosteroid medications, such as Prednisone, Cortisone, Prednisolone and Dexamethasone, are damaging to the bone. Other drugs that may increase the risk of osteoporosis include anti-depressants, Methotrexate, some breast cancer medications and some antibiotics.

Building Strong Bones

Once again I cannot help but emphasize on the importance of good nutrition in maintaining bone health. There are three key ingredients that we need to focus on for good bone health: protein, calcium and Vitamin-D. Although protein as a health-building block has been discussed extensively in this book, I am again going to touch upon it as it is a part of nutrition that can never be overstated.

Protein

The composition of the body changes after middle age, including an increase in the mass of fat and a decrease in lean mass (that is, muscle). One modifiable component of this process is dietary protein intake.

Protein from dairy and vegetable sources may not be complete in itself of all the required Amino acids, but protein complementing can take care of that. Protein must be a part of every meal and although there are various recommendations, an easy one to remember is 0.7-0.8 g/kg of body weight—so if you weigh 50 kg, your protein intake should be 35-40 g per day.

The best sources of protein are: lean chicken, fish, tofu and soya milk, beans, sprouts, eggs, dairy especially yoghurt, nuts and seeds (pumpkin, squash and watermelon seeds, peanuts, almonds).

Acid-Base Balance of the Diet

The impact of acid-base balance on bone is a comparatively new area of research. Your blood needs the right balance of acid and basic (alkaline) compounds to function properly. This is called the acid-base balance. Your kidneys and lungs work to keep the acid-base balance. Even slight variations from the normal range can have significant effects on your vital organs. To function properly, the body maintains the pH of blood close to 7.40. Investigation of the effect of ageing on blood acid-base composition suggests that reduced kidney function in older people diminishes the kidney's ability to excrete hydrogen ions in response to changes in blood pH. This disturbs the acid base balance and makes the blood more acidic as we grow older even in normal circumstances. So healthy adults manifest a low-grade, diet-dependent metabolic acidosis or acidic pH that increases with age.

Diet can contribute to acidosis when alkali-producing fruits and vegetables are consumed in insufficient amounts to balance the intake of acid-producing foods such as cereal grains and protein. The organic acids in fruits and vegetables are metabolized to alkaline bicarbonate; cereal grains contribute phytic and other acids and protein adds acid in proportion to its content of sulphur-containing Amino acids (which are metabolized to sulphuric acid).

An acidic environment has negative effects on preservation of bone in that it can impair bone-forming cells, activate bone resorption and exert a direct chemical effect on bone.

Calcium

Include plenty of calcium in your diet. For women between the ages of 19-50 and men between 19-70, the recommended dietary allowance (RDA) is 1000 milligrams (mg) of calcium a day. The recommendation increases to 1200 mg a day for women after the age of 50.

Good sources of calcium include dairy products, almond, broccoli, oatmeal, kale, canned salmon with bones, beans and legumes, sardines and soy products such as tofu. If you find it difficult to get enough calcium from your diet, ask your doctor about supplements.

Vitamin-D

Pay attention to Vitamin-D. Your body needs Vitamin-D to absorb calcium. For adults, both men and women, aged 19-70, the RDA of Vitamin-D is 600 international units (IUs) a day. The recommendation increases to 800 IUs a day for people aged 71 and older. International units are standardized measurements to be able to quantify and compare different formulations that provide the active vitamin. For example, Vitamin-D can be obtained from cod liver oil source or salmon source and calculating international units available in each of these sources helps us compare the better source or take the dosage accordingly.

Good sources of Vitamin-D include oily fish such as salmon, mackerel, tuna and sardines, cod liver oil, egg yolks, fortified cereals as in breakfast cereals which are supplemented and fortified by the addition of various vitamins according to recommendations, and orange juice, and fortified dairy products. Sunlight also contributes to the body's production of Vitamin-D. However it is an unreliable source. If you're worried about not getting enough Vitamin-D, ask your doctor for supplements.

Exercise

The importance of exercise towards building strong bones cannot be over emphasized. Moderate weight lifting under supervision, yoga and moderate cardio all help towards building strong bones and preventing osteoporosis.

Testing for Weak Bones

Both laboratory tests and X-rays may be done to evaluate for contributing factors. The most common blood tests measure the blood count, calcium and phosphorous, liver and kidney function, and thyroid level. Often a 24-hour urine collection is done to measure calcium. Other tests could be carried out depending on the circumstances. Previously unrecognized problems such as hyperthyroidism, hyperparathyroidism, celiac disease, hypercalciuria, and Cushing's Syndrome may be discovered.

In cases of fragile fractures or flat bone pain, consult a doctor, who will probably recommend a bone densitometry test. The results will help the doctor gauge your bone density and determine your rate of bone loss. By evaluating this information and your risk factors, they can assess whether you might be a candidate for medication to help slow bone loss.

Some of these bone problems may surface early in the form of twinges at the gym, or unexplained pain in certain awkward movements etc., but mostly these are asymptomatic. However it is absolutely essential to get your calcium, iron and D3 levels checked at periodic intervals if these pains continue to persist.

Tests for Bone Functioning

- Serum calcium
- Serum Vitamin-D3
- Blood count
- Liver function tests
- Renal function tests
- Hormone assay
- T3, T4, TSH
- Bone scan
- X-ray of suspected bones with CT if required
- Urine calcium (24-hours)

Medications

Medications are the last resort for osteoporosis. Although many are available, they all come with side effects and need to be administered only under strict medical supervision.

Remember that osteoporosis is typically the prototype disease approach to women's wellness. This means approaching it from a holistic approach of prevention, early diagnosis, lifestyle modifications and finally medication and intervention go a long way in making a lasting difference. Early care, exercise, healthy nutrition and lifestyle modifications build strong bones in addition to a healthy body. They can go a long way in preventing osteoporosis as we grow older.

TO SUMMARIZE

Bones can get fragile with age

Testing for calcium, Vitamin-D3 and bone density vital

A diet rich in calcium, Vitamin-D3, protein and amino acids necessary to keep the bones strong

Have vitamin and mineral supplements in your 40s

Exercise regularly

16

Positively Healthy

Rani is a 33-year-old software professional. She comes to my clinic every month for a peel and a chat. I look forward to her visits as she is always cheerful, ready for a quick laugh and unfailingly bright and optimistic. Rani is an ovarian cancer survivor. She struggles with various hormonal balance issues due to the surgery she underwent. Her face used to break out with acne and folliculitis, she grew facial hair where she had none before, her weight soared up but she remained cheerful through it all. And slowly but surely every one of her problems came under control with minimal medication but just with her positive attitude and unfailing good humour.

We often hear of examples of those who smile through adversity, those who conquered illnesses with good attitudes, but sometimes all of this tend to read like mere anecdotes far removed from reality. Sometimes the sheer magnitude of the problems we deal with seems to faze us completely. It seems like the universe is against us and there is little we can do to influence that in any manner.

Take a moment, pause and check with yourself. How is

your body feeling right at this moment? How is your mind feeling? Are you generally healthy? Do you feel something is not okay? Go step by step and check for subtle symptoms: Is your neck feeling tense? Does your lower back ache? Do you have a headache? Are you exhausted and irritable again? Perhaps you're battling a more serious health diagnosis and you're experiencing symptoms from your health condition.

Whether you're experiencing the nuisance of a minor physical symptom or the more worrying stress of a serious health condition, there is enough scientific evidence to show how the mind can actually assist actively in the process of healing with just the right response from the body. I am going to elaborate a bit more on this.

Self-healing

Our bodies are beautifully equipped with natural self-repair mechanisms that are under the influence of thoughts, feelings and beliefs that originate in our mind. It knows how to kill cancer cells, fix broken proteins, slow ageing, eliminate toxins, fight infections, get rid of foreign bodies, and otherwise keep us healthy. It also knows how to support treatments that we take to ensure that we get maximum results from the therapies we undergo. But more often than not, things go awry and diseases manifest themselves when these self-repair mechanisms fail to function properly.

Steps to a healthier you:

Get to the Root Cause of the Problem

I am not talking here about visiting the doctor and getting your diagnosis arising from the symptoms. You may be diagnosed with high blood pressure or a gall bladder cyst or a precancerous condition. But the diagnosis is just a medical confirmation of your problem. You need to dig deep into your mind to find out your feelings. What has been different? Have you been obsessing about something? Are your kids worrying you?

It is inevitable that each one of us will identify some trigger for stress that will underlie every symptom that we experience. But if everyone has stress, how is it that some people seem to sail through the toughest illnesses with a smile while others get bogged down by seemingly trifling issues?

Many scientists have looked at response to stress, its affect and its effect and some answers seem to be becoming clearer. Your nervous system has two operating systems, the 'fight-or-flight' stress response dominated by the sympathetic nervous system and the relaxation response run by the parasympathetic nervous system. Only when your nervous system is in a relaxed state does your body's self-repair mechanisms function!

So now the powers of introspection, meditation and relaxation seem to becoming a little clearer. The amygdala in the brain responds to stress with feelings of anxiety, fear and terror every single time. Our body triggers stress at least 50 times every day. If we do not train our mind to relax, we are triggering responses that inevitably lead to states of ill-being and disease.

Relax the mind. Learn and practise meditation and deep breathing and spending some quiet time with yourself every day to release the healing power of relaxation.

Cultivate Positive Relationships

It has again been proven scientifically that to foster healing and happiness, we need to be surrounded by a positive atmosphere and fulfilling relationships. Does this mean that how healthy we can be is driven by the people around us?

Of course not! It is our attitude which drives positivity in and around us. When people feel positive emotions, they feel closer and more connected to others around them. If one is thinking positively, they are more likely to make a favourable judgement about someone. For example, if a person in a negative frame of mind asks their friend to pick up some groceries on the way home from work but they forget something on the list, that person may get annoyed that their friend was forgetful and start an argument. However, someone with a positive outlook would have a different reaction: they'd probably thank their friend for making the effort to go to the supermarket after a long day at work and accept the item was forgotten due to tiredness rather than inconsiderateness. It would also make the friend feel positive about a good deed appreciated rather than that his or her faults are always picked on.

Sometimes, it is possible that people may constantly respond to you with negative inputs. At such times, it is wise to physically remove yourself from the scene till tempers cool down. Not being reactive is the first step to relaxation and can go a long way to keeping you healthy and well.

Listen to Your Body

Listen to your body and act accordingly. No one knows your body better than you. If something hurts, rest it. If you feel tired, take a break. If you feel you can push yourself to do a little extra work, do it. But learn to listen to your body and the body will listen to you and heal accordingly.

Work Hard, Rest Harder

We live in a world which rewards work and frowns on rest. However, rest drives relaxation which heals the mind and the body. Energy is not inexhaustible but needs to be replenished at regular intervals. Treat rest with as much respect as you treat work and watch your health and productivity increase.

Drop the Guilt

Guilt drives the most negative stress responses in the body. Guilt is also an exercise in futility as it is mostly about things past. Rehashing that only creates further stressful feelings in the body. This often leads to illness and drives feelings of isolation.

If there is something that you have done that troubles you, first accept that it has happened. Then look at your behavioural traits and see what you can try change so the situation does not occur again. This positive exercise itself will make you feel better and more positive and ultimately promote a sense of well-being.

Write a Healing Note

There is great healing power in writing. Write down your thoughts and feelings. Write down your negativities and fears. Then write the one thing that can help you feel better. And write that every day and write what steps you have taken to head in that direction. This is your healing note, your self-prescription to wellness. And it will work, without fail, every time!

Work towards Happiness

Most people set goals. They may be goals for wealth, achievements, career advancement, etc. Very few people write goals for happiness. It may be simple things: a lunch with your girlfriends, a walk with your dog, a movie with your daughter or just about anything. If you make it a goal, you will make it happen. Ultimately a state of wellness is not just a clean chit from your doctor; it is you feeling the wellness within yourself and your happiness spilling over to positively influence every aspect of your life.

Health and wellness form the cornerstone of a long, successful and happy life. It is increasingly clear to scientists that diagnosis and treatment form the smallest part of the journey to wellness. Each one of us is responsible for ensuring and delivering health and happiness to our individual selves, and for creating healthy families and communities. Women play the largest role in the health chain. A little bit more focus on us, our needs and our health and happiness outcomes can go a long way towards creating healthier and happier families, communities, nations and ultimately a healthy, happy world. Start today, in tiny ways that count, by taking control of your jelly bellies in whatever form or shape they may be, to correct what is disturbing your state of well-being.

Bringing It Together

I have emphasized, time and again in this book, the diversity of roles women play in today's world. Steeped in the business of getting on and staying on the carousel, a lot of 'ME' things get forgotten. Health should *never* be one of them.

Whatever you do at any point in your life, bring it all together to centre on your health and well-being. Focus on the four pillars that I mentioned in the first chapter and use them as a lens to work through every issue you face. Take the JB test once in six months after you have implemented these changes, and watch your JB index reduce and your health quotient increase.

Pay special attention to nutrition. Challenge yourself by creating healthy and tasty foods. Convert others into healthy eaters; make healthy and tasty foods a way of life.

Use your friends and support groups effectively. Actively help women around you in their quest for well-being. There is great power in the collectiveness of women. Harness it to drive wellness in you and around you.

Be positive in everything you do. Positivity promotes healing, cures diseases, and restores a state of harmony. Harness that harmony into your system.

Get healthy, stay well, and be happy!

Acknowledgements

My family for all the support and patience in tolerating my many moods during the writing of this book. Thank you Narayana, Sharan, Rajesh and Rocco for just being there.

My parents and brother for the constant encouragement and the cheerleading throughout my life! Thank you Amma, Appa and Murali.

My BFF Anjali Tendulkar for her presence in my life, her grace and dignity and her amazing focus on fitness and health among all the other things she means to me. She has taught me the need to prioritize oneself and I'm hoping all the readers will learn it too.

My dear friend Sachin Tendulkar for all the support with the book launch and for the lovely blurb for the book.

My dearest mentor and guide, Annabel Mehta, for all the wisdom and empathy that I have seen and try to learn from, while interacting in Apnalaya and various other forums. Thank you Anniemummy for everything!

My lovely married family, nieces and nephew who think I am capable of anything and everything!

My teachers, Dr Satish Wadhwa, Dr Uday Khopkar, Dr Rajiv Joshi, Dr V.V. Karkare, for the learnings, wisdom and encouragement.

My dearest agent and friend, Priya Doraswamy, for being the moving force in all my writing endeavours. Pri, may the laughter and fun never stop.

My editor, Debasri Rakshit, who I'm sure must have pulled out at least a few hairs in the course of this book. Thank you, lovely Deb, for never saying so and for believing that I have more books in me!

Sunayna Saraswat from HarperCollins for patiently reading the proofs, correcting errors and offering valuable suggestions to make the content look better.

The entire team at HarperCollins India, the editorial team, the art department and the marketing and sales teams and all the other lovely people. Thank you, all of you, for everything!

The Saffola team at Marico, especially Minakshi, Avik and Anshul, for sharing all the research and for the commitment to improving heart health of women.

My young and hardworking research assistant, Neha Sawant, for all her help with the background research for this book. Thank you, Neha, for your diligence and patience in dealing with all my demands.

My friend, Manoj Warrier, for his wisdom and his help whenever I need it! Thank you, Manoj, for all the help with this book and elsewhere.

My girl gang, Rujuta, Chitra, Devika, Sheela and Kamala for all the laughs and insights. Thank you lovely ladies! A special thank you to Kamala for the feedback on the proofs and my yoga teacher, Sangeeta for suggesting the asanas.

All the women I have worked with, had fun with, at the beauty pageants, at my clinic, at Apnalaya, at all the forums I speak in and everywhere else, you have inspired this book. Thank you for making it possible!